T0374349

A LEADERSHIP TOOLKIT FOR NURSES AND HEALTHCARE PROFESSIONALS

This practical guide provides essential knowledge and tools for nursing and healthcare students and practitioners to develop their leadership skills, from the very beginning of their practice and throughout their careers.

The first section provides an overview of leadership in nursing and healthcare in today's context, discussing:

- relevant theory, and values-based approaches such as congruent, compassionate and ethical leadership;
- the role of nurses and healthcare professionals in policy, social justice and decision making, and how leadership positively impacts quality of patient care and the healthcare professions;
- how we learn leadership skills, such as emotional and social intelligence, and experiential methods of learning, such as reflexivity, learning from experience and Action Learning.

The second section looks at the role of emotions and experiential learning in leadership development, and methods such as action learning, reflexivity, lifelong journaling and the use of narratives and the arts, to introduce a range of practical tools and methods for the reader to use in their own development. Strategies for the less experienced practitioner and for the more experienced practitioner are presented, including action learning and promoting wellbeing, and the book also highlights the evidence base the methods draw on. This creative text introduces vital tools and uses reflective activities and questions to support readers in building their leadership skills.

It is ideal for students and practitioners at all levels in nursing and healthcare interested in self-development.

Alison H. James is a Doctor of Advanced Healthcare Practice and is currently Reader in Healthcare Leadership at Cardiff University, UK and a Senior Fellow of the Higher Education Academy (HEA). She is a Registered Nurse with a background in neurosciences, critical care, osteoporosis and clinical research. Alison has taught across undergraduate and postgraduate healthcare programmes for over 20 years, has published and worked on leadership development projects internationally, and is an active qualitative researcher. Alison's main interests are in research on leadership development and education in the healthcare workforce and how this impacts delivery and quality of patient care, with a focus on values-based leadership theory and models, and how this influences cultures within healthcare environments.

A LEADERSHIP TOOLKIT FOR NURSES AND HEALTHCARE PROFESSIONALS

From Student to Experienced Practitioner

Alison H. James

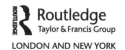

Routledge
Taylor & Francis Group

LONDON AND NEW YORK

Designed cover image: Getty Images

First published 2025
by Routledge
4 Park Square, Milton Park, Abingdon, Oxon OX14 4RN

and by Routledge
605 Third Avenue, New York, NY 10158

Routledge is an imprint of the Taylor & Francis Group, an informa business

© 2025 Alison H. James

The right of Alison H. James to be identified as author of this work has been asserted in accordance with sections 77 and 78 of the Copyright, Designs and Patents Act 1988.

All rights reserved. No part of this book may be reprinted or reproduced or utilised in any form or by any electronic, mechanical, or other means, now known or hereafter invented, including photocopying and recording, or in any information storage or retrieval system, without permission in writing from the publishers.

Trademark notice: Product or corporate names may be trademarks or registered trademarks, and are used only for identification and explanation without intent to infringe.

British Library Cataloguing-in-Publication Data
A catalogue record for this book is available from the British Library

ISBN: 978-1-032-56011-3 (hbk)
ISBN: 978-1-032-56010-6 (pbk)
ISBN: 978-1-003-43335-4 (ebk)

DOI: 10.4324/9781003433354

Typeset in Baskerville
by codeMantra

CONTENTS

ABOUT THE AUTHOR

Alison H. James

Alison is a Doctor of Advanced Healthcare Practice and is currently Reader in Healthcare Leadership at Cardiff University, UK and a Senior Fellow of the Higher Education Academy (HEA). She is a Registered Nurse with a background in neurosciences, critical care, osteoporosis, and clinical research. Alison has taught across undergraduate and postgraduate healthcare programmes for over 20 years, has published and worked on leadership development projects internationally, and is an active qualitative researcher. Her main interests are in research on leadership development and education in the healthcare workforce and how this impacts delivery and quality of patient care, with a focus on values-based leadership theory and models, and how this influences cultures within healthcare environments.

NOTES ON CONTRIBUTORS

Clare Bennett

Dr Bennett is a Registered Nurse with a background in sexual health, immunology, HIV and infectious diseases. She is a Doctor of Nursing and is currently a Reader at Cardiff University, UK. She has taught leadership, quality improvement, and patient safety on undergraduate and postgraduate programmes for nurses and allied health professionals for over two decades in the UK and throughout Europe. She has also researched and written about leadership internationally. Clare is co-director of the Wales Centre for Evidence Based Care in Cardiff, and teaches and coaches in the field of evidence development and implementation.

Mandy Brimble

Mandy is a Doctor of Advanced Healthcare Practice, a Reader in Children and Young People's Nursing, and Senior Fellow of Advance HE. She is also a Registered Children's Nurse and Health Visitor. She has worked in a range of clinical settings and was lead practitioner for education and research at Tŷ Hafan children's hospice in Wales, where she now serves as a member of the Clinical Governance Committee. She has undertaken many roles at Cardiff University School of Healthcare Sciences, including Director for Undergraduate Studies with responsibility for 2,000 students registered on nine undergraduate programmes across nursing and allied health professions. Her publication profile encompasses a range of professional journals and joint editorship of a book entitled *Nursing Care of Children and Young People with Long-Term Conditions* (Brimble & McNee, 2021). She is associate editor of the *Journal of Child Health Care* and chair of the All-Wales Paediatric Palliative Care Education and Training Group. She is also a member of the International Children's Palliative Care Network and an Education Committee member of the International Family Nursing Association. Her interest in emotional and social intelligence stems from her doctoral work examining emotional labour and professional integrity in children's hospices. Mandy has recently been commissioned to write a book on emotional labour in children's nursing.

Teena J. Clouston

Teena J Clouston is a Professor Emerita in Occupational Therapy and Wellbeing at Cardiff University, UK. Her research and scholarly activity consider the interrelationships of socio-political/cultural constructs and values on health and wellbeing. In this context, she is intrigued by the influence of neoliberal principles on achieving life balance, wellbeing, and personal meaning in life. While this tends to focus on the neoliberal drives for intensification, performativity, and increased individualism, responsibility and accountability in the paid workplace, Professor Clouston also considers the impact of these forces in terms of connections at multiple levels, such as family, community and relationships with the natural world. In particular, her work has highlighted how individuals cope with these pressures by compromising personally meaningful activities, and thus wellbeing, in order to prioritise completing the everyday, obligatory tasks people feel they *have to do* in order to successfully get through their over-busy lives. Professor Clouston is also intrigued by the challenges of learning and teaching caring and compassionate values in health and social care professions, how these translate into personal wellbeing in everyday practice, and how this can be sustained or otherwise through implementing values-based leadership in challenging organisational settings.

PREFACE

I was a newly qualified nurse in the first year of registration in 1989 when I realised that understanding leadership was important for my career in nursing. I was shadowing the ward sister in the clinical area when I became aware of something very subtle yet powerful in her interaction with the medical teams and her advocacy for patients and staff. This fascinated me. What I was observing was an example of a highly emotionally intelligent professional demonstrating an authentic approach to leadership with clarity and confidence. This is one example of how observing mentors in practice became important in my development as a nurse and my future career as I became more and more aware of the skills and effects of both effective and ineffective leadership. I also began to appreciate the importance of effective leadership within healthcare and its effects on the culture of work environments and on standards of patient care. Studying the concepts, aspects, and many connotations of 'leadership' has allowed me to observe with fascination the nuances, impact and possibilities.

More recently I have been fortunate to be able to really delve deeper into the implications of leadership in all its forms through research and study and in discussions with my students, which has only driven further my interest in its power to be a positive and negative force within organisations. I would propose that, as healthcare professionals, we need to gain a deep understanding of our own personal leadership approach and realise its effects on those we communicate with, work with and provide care for. We also have a responsibility as professionals in healthcare to be leaders for our professions. Without a clear understanding of what leadership means in this context and how it is practised, we cannot fully meet the requirements of our professional obligations. We may not all gain positional leadership or positions in the hierarchy of organisations; and indeed not all wish to follow that career path. However, all can lead, influence and shape healthcare practice, champion the standards of care provided and influence the cultures and teamwork in our working contexts. If you are reading this book, I assume you are passionate about your career, and, to quote Craig et al. from Chapter 4, we take the view here that "leadership is a choice, not a title" (2015, p. xi).

In this book we aim to inform, inspire and support nurses and care professionals in both understanding and developing their own approach to personal leadership. As a useful resource, it presents an overview of why leadership is important in healthcare, and introduces tools and techniques for developing an incremental approach to personal leadership over the course of a career. From undergraduate level through to post-registration, to nurses and healthcare professionals who are more experienced and are interested in developing their leadership skills, approaches to developing methods that are helpful at all stages are presented. This is a contemporary text exploring current thinking and challenging leadership while introducing creative approaches to self-development as well as methods to apply in practice. In teaching leadership and quality improvement I have used visual images, metaphors and symbolism for many years. I have found that students engage with the process and often express how they can dip into the 'toolbox' of methods as they progress. The methods explored here include visual thinking strategies and exercises to start you on your path to exploring this creative approach.

We know that healthcare globally faces challenges in the workforce in attracting and retaining professionals in their chosen specialities. There are many reasons for this attrition; however many feel limited by their lack of influence or power over the shaping of healthcare provision and their inability to contribute and influence decisions. There are also powerful historical legacies within some healthcare organisations and professions that have negative influences on how we perceive leadership and levels of power. However evidence in the healthcare literature demonstrates the value of highly skilled, effective and influential clinical-level nurses and executive-level nurse leaders who contributed to key decision making and leadership during the COVID-19 pandemic. While there are many courses and opportunities for healthcare professionals to develop leadership skills following registration, there remains a disparity in expectations and the reality for students.

When exploring perceptions of leadership with student nurses, my colleagues and I have found that student nurses rarely viewed their role as involving leadership, and many felt unprepared to lead within the profession. Although nurses in the United Kingdom are expected to demonstrate leadership at the point of registration, there remains a disparate approach to leadership education and preparation, and this is common across professions. As with many skills in life, leadership requires a long-term view, so consider it as a companion along your path of professional development – something you learn from and cultivate constantly. Expect your leadership to change as you progress as a professional and as your self-reflection develops. Be thoughtful and contemplative of your own leadership and how it is perceived by others, and be observant of how others lead. When you experience negative leadership examples, explore the detail and use your critical thinking skills to understand the detail and nuances of why, what and how.

Developing an approach to leadership is a continuous, incremental and often career-spanning journey of personal growth. There are many resources from a variety of disciplines that analyse and debate the aspects of success and the known pitfalls of differing leadership approaches. From historical perspectives and social influences, exploring the changing features of leadership theories provides a fascinating insight into changing values, societal norms and global events that influence these changes. Historical theories are therefore important to how we view both personal leadership development and how we see leadership portrayed by others. Indeed, leadership is often used interchangeably with 'management', or is combined in one sentence within organisational strategies and even development courses. The focus of this book is individual leadership, drawing on newer developing theories of leadership, defining the importance of personal and professional values, and using creative approaches to critical reflection to gain self-insight. Many 'quick-fix' tools can be found with a brief internet search, based on personality types and tendencies that can provide a snapshot view. This book aims to be the antithesis. Rather than a shortcut to leadership, it aims to be a companion which will be useful across the career, and provides methods that can become positive habit-forming approaches to self-insight for leadership. It should be acknowledged that individuals' career trajectories differ: while some will seek to take positional leadership positions and become organisationally focused, others will not. In both instances, self-insight is valuable, and being able to connect, inspire and motivate others requires the ability to question and challenge self-perception and recognise how actions and words impact others. Effective leadership can make a genuine contribution to improving patient care and making the health service more robust and responsive for patients.

The book is presented in two parts. In Part 1 we explore leadership, its importance in healthcare, and past and present leadership theories, moving through aspects of leadership such as emotional intelligence, change, developing personal leadership and the importance of wellbeing. In Part 2 we present some methods and tools for development, including creative methods.

Chapter 1 explores why leadership is important in nursing and healthcare, and provides an overview of some of the more recent values-based leadership theories. Chapter 2 explores leadership during crises and in challenging times. Within healthcare, we know effective leadership is essential for addressing challenges that sometimes arise, so learning from examples of crises and challenges is important. Areas that have emerged from the evidence, including moral distress and emotional labour, along with the possibilities of positive disruptive leadership, are addressed. In Chapter 3 I introduce issues of power, politics and social justice, exploring how you can be heard and exert influence at a local and wider level, along with a discussion of some of the challenges for healthcare professionals. Chapter 4 considers areas that are helpful to consider across your career and your personal leadership development, such as empowerment and what it means for you and the choices you make. Generational differences are briefly discussed as we know the formative years of our lives shape our views and motivation in our careers and working lives. The importance of role models and emotions is also considered as they inform our leadership learning and development. Chapter 5 provides a clear overview of the components of social and emotional intelligence, their similarities and differences. Different types of empathy are outlined, together with the importance of using cognitive and compassionate empathy, not emotional empathy, in professional caring relationships. Social and emotional intelligence is essential in a healthcare career. It underpins all interpersonal interactions and is especially important for effective, compassionate leadership at every stage of a career. Chapter 6 sets out some key leadership strategies to enable you to effectively lead change and support others throughout the process of change. It will also help you question whether a proposed change will lead to an improvement in care delivery and to understand why some people are resistant to change. Chapter 7 explores the nature of wellbeing and how that can be sustained within leadership roles, particularly in health and social care settings. A brief overview of the challenges for leaders in these setting is discussed, followed by an introduction to some practical techniques and tools that can be used to support leaders and their staff to achieve and maintain their own wellbeing at work and in everyday life.

Part 2 begins with a return to emotional intelligence, and Chapter 8 revisits the concepts of social and emotional intelligence outlined in Chapter 5, gives an overview of how these skills can be developed, and uses a case study to demonstrate how leaders can use social and emotional intelligence in challenging situations. Interactive activities will help the reader explore how leadership is underpinned by emotional and social intelligence skills at key points in 'Jenny's' career, from being a student to becoming an experienced practitioner. Alternative approaches to each situation are also considered. Chapter 9 builds on the concept of professional and personal values, which we introduced in the first part of the book and further in Chapter 2. Suggested exercises and methods of exploring values and ethics, and what they mean for leadership, are offered. Chapter 10 takes us back to reflection and how creative methods such as journaling, visual thinking strategies and storytelling can support leadership development over time. Finally, in Chapter 11 we consider 'Action Learning' and how this method can be helpful both for personal leadership development and to support teams and problem solving in practice. I hope you find this book helpful in your leadership development.

Alison H. James

ACKNOWLEDGEMENTS

I would like to thank all our students who have been enthusiastic and committed to developing their knowledge and experience in healthcare. A special thank goes to all those who participated in our varied research that underpins much of this book, having given their time to enable the building of new knowledge from their own experiences. I am indebted to the contributors, valued colleagues who generously gave their time and commitment to completing the chapters, and without whom I could not have produced this book: Dr Clare L. Bennett, Dr Mandy Brimble and Professor Emerita Teena Clouston. Thanks also to my previous co-writers of books and articles, including David Stanley, who generously took me on the journey of writing – a truly great mentor. I also thank and appreciate all the healthcare professionals and academic colleagues who have contributed to my own experiences and understanding of leadership, healthcare, education and research over many years. I must include my mother, Mrs Valerie James, in this as an inspiring Registered Nurse and District Nurse with many years' experience who ignited my passion for both nursing and leadership, and provided me with tales of her nursing career to draw on. I would also like to extend a very special thank you to Bethan Kitson, a talented visual merchandiser who supported me with visual images and designed the 'Values Tree'.

This book has relied on the support of the publication team at Routledge/Taylor & Francis, and I am grateful for their continued encouragement. There are many more students and colleagues who have contributed to driving my interest and seeking new areas to explore in the constantly shifting and evolving enigma of leadership. Thank you.

Alison H. James

PART 1

CHAPTER 1

AN INTRODUCTION TO LEADERSHIP

Alison H. James

1.1 INTRODUCTION

This chapter will explore definitions of leadership and the importance of leadership in nursing and healthcare. A brief overview of traditional leadership theories is provided as a background. While historical approaches to leadership are important to provide context, in this book we will focus on more current values-based leadership theories. Over many centuries, writers, academics, and philosophers have explored the complexities and characteristics of leadership, trying to understand both the positive and negative influences and the impact of leadership on others. This exploration is still relevant to healthcare professionals and to our current healthcare system. It is relevant because we need to know how our own approach to leadership, and that of others, can impact and influence our professions and the care we provide to patients.

As healthcare professionals who work within complex healthcare systems, we believe in the importance of providing individuals with the best care possible, and so it is essential that we understand the dynamics and subtleties that influence this care. For most healthcare professionals, patients are always at the centre of our decision making, and we have professional values that we align with in our professional practice. Anything that influences the care we deliver is worth further consideration, and sometimes further scrutiny. For example, you may come across leaders who you consider are not exhibiting behaviours and attitudes that align with your professional values. This may cause ethical and moral challenges. Being self-aware and confident of the values that are central to the profession and to your own leadership philosophy can help with these challenging dilemmas. We will explore this further in Chapter 9. Identifying leadership styles and behaviours in others is also helpful to fully understand what, and sometimes why, these are being applied.

All healthcare professionals have an influence on the delivery of care. All are highly skilled and bring expertise from particular professional areas to create an individualised, evidence-based, carefully considered interprofessional care service for patients. Therefore, all are leaders within the healthcare context, whatever their position in the organisation. Trying to describe or understand leadership is not simple or straightforward. However, exploring it further and really understanding its possibilities, both positive and negative, makes it much more of an interesting topic to explore, practise, and develop in a professional and personal capacity.

While leadership in all healthcare professions has developed through history, nursing has an interesting backdrop as its professional origins are based on models of servitude, subservience, and self-sacrifice to the medical profession. Hierarchy and power dynamics have been present throughout its history, and still are to some extent as healthcare services, while modernised in some respects, continue to exert traditional structures of hierarchy (James & Bennett 2022). For many years, leadership was not something seriously considered relevant to Nursing and Allied Health educational curricula. This is changing, although it remains one of those contentious skills that compete with clinical skills in already full curricula, and is often confused with aspects of management, often misunderstood and sometimes idealised. While researching student nurses' and academics' experiences of leadership in my own research, it was clear that

DOI: 10.4324/9781003433354-2

not all student nurses felt leadership was part of their role, and felt underprepared from both their higher education and their clinical experience and learning as students (James et al. 2022).

Reflective Activity: 1.1

Think about your understanding of leadership. Firstly, think of some global leaders or figures from history.

> Do you consider any of them to be a great leader, and if so, why?
>
> What qualities made them effective or ineffective leaders? Write these down.
>
> Now think about leaders you have come across in the healthcare context, of any profession.
>
> What qualities made them effective or ineffective leaders? Write these down.

Reflect on the qualities you have identified in the reflection above. For both categories, effective and ineffective, consider how leadership impacts the delivery of patient care, teamwork, and the wider organisation.

1.2   HOW WE DEFINE LEADERSHIP AND LEARN TO BE LEADERS

Definitions of leadership are wide-ranging and sometimes are more relevant to specific disciplines. However, many theorists agree that leaders influence and exert influence over others to accomplish their desired goals or aims (Stogdill 1948, Northouse 2007, Grossman & Valiga 2021). Leadership can also be viewed as accomplishing aims with the support of others (Leigh & Maynard 1995). The perspective of leadership as an influencing force acknowledges that people without formal power or not in formal positions can be leaders. This means that leadership can be learned and developed whatever your role, and this contradicts traditional concepts of leadership, which viewed it as a skill one is born with.

Some leadership theorists identify leaders as effecting change (Kotter 1990, pp. 37–60), as influencing people into taking action and therefore creating agency for change, rather than being agents of stability and constancy (Bennis & Nanus 1985). This can also help clarify the differences between management and leadership, as managers need to strive for stability, order and minimal risk to maintain the status quo and keep things working. Leaders however are sometimes risk takers and visionaries, creating conditions for innovation and movement.

As leadership thinking has developed and research into leadership has evolved, there is now further concentration on the importance of relationships and attending to values within groups and teams, rather than on leadership being power-based and positional. Finding meaning and basing actions on principles has become more popular in the literature (Stanley 2022); and, while personal leadership remains a focus of leadership theories, there has been a shift from the egotistical self-centredness of achieving positional leadership to the impact on the followers and the organisations in which a leader functions and belongs.

Leadership has become more about selecting and aligning with values, articulating and demonstrating those values through appropriate actions, and developing a vision for followers. Greenfield describes this as "a wilful act where one person attempts to construct the social world for others ... leaders will try to commit others to the values that they themselves believe are good" (1986, p. 166). This is especially important currently within healthcare and its professions as all are heavily entrenched in values and principles. If we consider the importance of leadership on organisational cultures, then leaders set the tone, the boundaries, and the aims, and establish the acceptable and unacceptable standards of practice within an organisation or team. Even in the world of business there has been a shift towards the more values-based styles as evidence emerges of their effects on workforces and wellbeing.

Since the COVID-19 pandemic, the issue of workforce and wellbeing has raised further concern for leaders in healthcare, including the effects of multiple sources of stress placed on workers (Couarraze et al. 2021). Writers and researchers are responding with recommendations for more empathetic, compassionate, and ethical approaches to leadership (West 2021). However, there is a risk that these may oversimplify matters and become idealised rhetoric rather than useful approaches that consider and address the complex nature of the many issues facing organisations (James et al. 2023). Indeed, as highly qualified and skilled professionals, we in healthcare are ideally placed and equipped to question and apply a critical eye to leadership theories and trends. While new, ethical, and values-based leadership approaches emerge in response to the societal, economic and global conditions we are confronted with, it is important to remind ourselves of the skills and potential available to us to support our development as effective leaders for patients and for colleagues we work with.

As you build your own personal approach to leadership, it is important to acknowledge and tap into your experience and knowledge and appreciate fully how this can support your leadership development. In the second part of this book, we present some helpful tools and methods that you can take through your career and apply. However, first it is helpful to set out briefly the different types of learning, experience, and knowledge. These are important for leadership development and allow further criticality and reflexivity as we approach the theory and place importance on experience of leadership. For example, from my own research with student nurses, many spoke of the impact mentors had on their ideas of what type of leader they would like to be in the future; however, if they lacked opportunities to reflect on this, they felt learning opportunities had been lost (James et al. 2022). Many also felt that what they learned in university didn't align with what they experienced in practice, so the links between theory, evidence, and practice are important in many aspects of the learning experience and in learning about leadership. Combining *tacit*, *implicit* and *explicit* knowledge can really impact and form your leadership profile and leadership *mastery*, and we will further explore learning and development in Chapter 5 (Henriksen & Børgesen 2016, James et al. 2024b).

- **Tacit knowledge** includes experience, skills, personal wisdom, and insight, rooted in context and time. During challenging times, this knowledge from experience is embedded and unique, and can be an important source for future learning. However, it is sometimes difficult to share and express. For example, a nursing student may observe an experienced nurse during a clinical emergency. If the experienced nurse does not sit with the student and allow questions to be asked – critical reflection, rationale for actions, and links to an evidence base – the tacit knowledge may remain as observational and surface learning for the student.

- **Implicit knowledge** is sometimes confused with tacit knowledge; however it is subtly different as it can form a link between tacit and explicit knowledge. Implicit knowledge represents subconscious understanding, or assumptions that individuals may not immediately be aware of. Through reflection and deeper thinking, it can become written and documented and an important step for translating experience into future learning. For example, encouraging students to write down critical reflection following clinical experience provides deeper experiential learning, and can be shared through conscious mentoring and socialisation.

- **Explicit knowledge** is codified recorded knowledge such as documented data and information, for example patient records and information technology (IT) data, and is more conceptualised.

Reflective Activity: 1.2

Think about an experience of seeing others leading; this could be a mentor or someone you have worked with in an area of clinical practice. How did the professional lead the situation? How were decisions made?

Reflect on what kind of leadership behaviours were exhibited. Was the leader direct and certain? Did they collaborate and share the decision making? Were they hesitant or uncertain?

Did you have an opportunity to discuss the decision making and approach with that person, and would it have helped? What would you have done in that situation?

Leadership is a complex process with multiple dimensions (Northouse 2007, Jones & Bennett 2018), and therefore there is no right or wrong definition. Organisations may have clear expectations of their leaders in what they should do and how they should behave; but there is much more opportunity and scope for individuals to carve out individualised concepts from the plethora of leadership literature, and to create a personal vision for individual leadership development to realise those expectations. The following definition is suggested by James and Stanley (2024, p. 24) within the context of leadership in nursing, but I would suggest this can apply to all healthcare professions, and particularly in terms of personal leadership: "Unifying people around core values and then constructing the social world around those values, inspiring innovation and helping people get through change."

1.3 THEORIES OF LEADERSHIP

Many leadership theories have emerged from business and other disciplines; and, while in this book we are mainly concerned with individual and personal leadership development, we are also concerned with the evidence for effective leadership and the principles and values that shape our professions. Many writers and academics have tried to fiercely advocate for the importance of leadership in healthcare and its impact on patient safety and standards of care. However, its popularity sometimes leads to simplification and to being viewed as a panacea, without recognition of the complexity of healthcare organisations and the workforce. As James et al. state in their call to rethink idealised nursing leadership, "The leadership industry has become a juggernaut that is seemingly unstoppable, with an ever-increasing audience seeking to become better leaders" (2024b, p. 8). Clark and Thompson (2022) are also sceptical of what they term the 'leadership illusion', so it is both wise and professional to consider with criticality what the evidence tells us about leadership within the context of our practice. While theories can provide background and ideas, it is important to also consider what theories support our professional values and can be evidenced as effective or demonstrated to support the realities of the complex and challenging contexts of healthcare.

Understanding the history of leadership theory is important for many reasons. It provides us with a view across the social and historical contexts that shape their development and inform us about how and why we view and interpret 'leadership' as it is today. Current theories have developed from, been influenced by, and are a reaction to older concepts. Also, while some of these may not be fully embraced as ideal leadership approaches now, and seem outdated, you may come across individuals who continue to lead in this way, and indeed circumstances where a more traditional approach is more effective. Therefore, as part of your own leadership development, it is good to gain an understanding of these styles. Below is a brief overview of the main theories, and we will focus further on more current values-based theories throughout the book.

The great man theory

Linked to religious and power connotations, this theory suggested that leadership was a birthright or given by divine command, and also linked to lineage and often class structure (Galton 1869, Man 2010, Bennis & Nanus 1985, Khan et al. 2016). This theory is discredited by historical examples of leaders being effective from all backgrounds, and any gender and level of society (Stanley et al. 2022).

Charismatic heroes

Lowney (2003) suggests that charismatic leadership relies on principles of self-awareness, ingenuity, love, and heroism. While we can identify examples today of charismatic leadership, this form is often linked to goal setting and individual heroism.

The big bang theory

This theory appeared in the wake of the calamitous events of the late nineteenth and early twentieth century. It suggests that leaders emerge from significant events or circumstances. Examples from history and politics, and more recently the COVID-19 pandemic, can be used to demonstrate examples of this: Abraham Lincoln emerged from the events of mid nineteenth-century America to lead his country; Boris Johnson rose through the divisions in the UK during the Brexit period; and Jacinda Ardern, although already an elected leader in New Zealand, gained further prominence globally during the pandemic when she demonstrated a caring and honest leadership style, gaining public support and praise. Stanley et al. (2022), however, make the interesting argument that this theory discounts the foundational work and preparation many of these leaders have done prior to the significant event, which undoubtedly prepared them in some way. In clinical practice, many nurse leaders adapted their approach to leadership during the pandemic; and, from the evidence, it is clear that, for some, this was a consolidation of their prior leadership experience – a challenge in adapting their approach that, at times, produced ethical dilemmas for them as professionals (James et al. 2024a).

Trait theory

Trait theory assumes that features and characteristics of the leader dominate situations, and many theorists have compiled lists of attributes they believe leaders possess (Mann 1959, Stogdill 1948, Grossman & Valiga 2021). However, this theory neglects the context of leading (Northouse 2007) and the personality of the individual (Mann 1959).

Style theories

These include laissez-faire, democratic, paternalistic, autocratic and/or dictatorial leadership (Handy 1999, Lett 2002, Northouse 2007). They offer some thoughts on the style used by the leader and are more descriptive and behavioural. These theories can be useful when considering what style or approach is required; however they omit detail on values and core beliefs, offering a surface approach to leadership overall.

Situational or contingency theory

Both situational and contingency theories develop further insight into the reasons and responses of leadership situations, and what impacted on the success of some leadership approaches. Many researchers – including Fiedler (1967), Tannenbaum and Schmidt (1958), Vroom and Yetton (1973), and Hersey and Blanchard (1988) – have suggested that effectiveness depended on the relationships between the aims, the leader's interpersonal skills and the context. Handy (1999) suggested that followers' trust and respect for the leader, the power status of the leader and the clarity of objectives are all elements that influence the success of the leader. These facets of followers' perceptions of leadership effectiveness have recently emerged as important in the wider evidence of general leadership during the pandemic (James et al. 2024a). However, Stanley et al. (2022) suggest that both theories are considered more managerial and human-resource focused overall.

Transactional leadership theory

Jones and Bennett (2018) describe transactional leaders as focusing on the principles and needs of the organisation, and directing people to do what is needed to achieve the desired outcomes through a reward and punishment approach. Transactional leaders manage day-to-day tasks to keep organisations in line with their functions (Burns 1978) and suggest a form of control and order. Criticism of this leadership approach includes an assumption that people are driven by rewards and punishments, and the inhibiting of innovation and creativity (Stanley et al. 2022). There are, however, some contexts where transactional leadership may be the most effective approach – for example, in military contexts and clinical emergencies as the rationale for this leadership approach is functionality and control of the context, limiting uncertainty and deviation from the desired state.

Transformational leadership theory

Distinguishing between management and leadership, this theory attempts to explore why some leaders can inspire followers in any situation (Northouse 2007). Bennis and Nanus (1985) suggested that transformational leadership links the process of paying attention to the needs of followers, and thereby increases motivation. Transformational leaders create a shared vision while maintaining enthusiasm and empowering others. These authors identified four themes central to this leadership theory – vision, communication, trust, and self-knowledge. By placing meaning on the work of others, the transformational leader is supportive, less hierarchical, and thus able to function at any level in an organisation. This allows for the leader to potentially change and improve areas and encourage innovative practice.

Authentic leadership

As a more recent theory, authentic leadership holds values, integrity and role modelling as important. Guided by passion and purpose, the authentic leader respects and listens to others, and has been associated with positive behaviours, reduced stress and greater retention in the nursing profession (Avolio & Gardner 2005, Wong & Cummings 2009). Being an authentic leader includes aligning people to a shared purpose, having a set of shared and united values, empowering others

---

Reflective Activity: 1.3

Think about leadership *styles* and reflect on the clinical area you work in now. What leadership style does the manager/team leader, apply?

You may want to consider some of the following styles that describe their approach:

Coaching, Directing, Delegating, Supporting, Charismatic, Participatory, Visionary, Pacesetting, Affirmative, Commanding, Inspiring, Autocratic.

Now consider examples of what actions and/or behaviours they demonstrate that have directed you to the chosen style.

What do you think are positive and/or negative aspects of this style?

Would you consider this to be an effective and positive role model for your leadership development? Why or why not?

---

to thrive, and being in contact and connecting effectively with others. Overall, authentic leaders pass on their skills and encourage others to develop their own authentic leadership style.

Servant leadership theory

Servant leadership reflects some the attributes of authentic leadership. Developed by Greenleaf (1977), the concept allows leaders to draw on trust collaboration, empathy, and ethical power as its main features, with less emphasis placed on hierarchy and position. Leaders are encouraged to 'serve' others while aligning with the organisation's aims and values (James et al. 2021, Jones & Bennett 2018). With a focus on involving and 'serving' patients and service users, this theory aligns with nursing and healthcare as an approach to develop and lead healthcare services. A study by Hanse et al. (2016) demonstrated that nurse managers who exhibited servant leadership developed effective relationships in their teams and supported organisations that valued the development of people. Criticism of the theory includes the language used, such as the term 'servant', and that it emphasises gender bias (Eicher-Catt 2005). However, this theory further shifts leadership towards the values-based approaches we now find emerging especially within healthcare contexts, with principles such as empathy, foresight, stewardship, and development at the centre.

Shared/collaborative leadership

Shared or collaborative leadership involves an approach which is contrary to the traditional approach of one person in the position of power. Rather, it encourages two or more individuals influencing the direction of teams to maximise effectiveness in a collaborative approach (Bergman et al. 2012). Other definitions include collaborative leaders applying appropriate skills and expertise, and 'distributing' these as the situation requires. 'Distributed leadership' moves away from positional leadership to other levels in an organisation through innovation and new practice, and 'system leadership' focuses on shared ambitions and goals rather than authority.

Congruent leadership

Stanley (2008) developed the congruent leadership theory following research into perspectives of clinical nurse leadership. From the lens of clinical practice this theory proposes a values-based approach which suggests *congruence* between actions and beliefs/values and the affinity felt by followers when a leader demonstrates these clearly, enabling and supporting follower commitment. Stanley's research (2008, 2019) identified clinically focused nurses and professionals who demonstrated values purposefully and clearly and expressed congruent leadership approaches. The clear demonstration of these values was evident to those they cared for and worked alongside, and demonstrated a congruent approach in leadership (James & Stanley 2024). Principles of congruent leadership include demonstrating emotional intelligence, compassionate engagement with others, visibility in practice, good communication, and role modelling for followers. As motivating influencers, congruent leaders clearly align actions to values in decision making and communication, and show passion and enthusiasm for their profession and practice.

Compassionate leadership

Michael West states that: "The purpose of compassionate leadership in health and social care is to help create the conditions where all those in our communities are supported to live the best and most fulfilling lives" (2021, p. 4). In developing a framework for leadership that places compassion at its centre, West takes the elements of compassion – attending, understanding, empathising and helping – and applies them to the contexts of leadership in health and social care. In acknowledgement of the crisis facing health and social care in the UK, he proposed that staff who are valued, listened to, and supported are more likely to thrive and contribute to the wisdom, humanity and high-quality of care within services. With a flattening of hierarchy and shared sense of responsibility through autonomy and respect, a compassionate leader promotes inclusion, creativity and improvement, creating stronger connectivity, raising levels of trust, and enhancing a collective approach to improving services for patients.

Hougaard et al. (2020) emphasise the importance of wisdom and leadership competence in this approach, and argue that compassion alone is insufficient. We know leadership is not easy; it requires making difficult and sometimes unpopular decisions, being brave, and having clarity of direction. To support these leadership requirements, Hougaard et al. suggest leaders need to be mindful and present, and aware of the emotions and behaviours of others. Compassionate leadership draws on several values-based theories, and de Zulueta (2015) suggests it lacks a clear theoretical underpinning. However, its focus on organisational culture and the role this plays in lapses of care and challenges for the future of healthcare services means it has gathered support, further research, and debate. In its positive approach, compassionate leadership addresses: connecting individual and organisational values; influencing organisational cultures, positive behaviours and role modelling supported by policies and structures within the organisation; and demonstrating kindness, honesty and transparency along with courage in challenging behaviours when needed (Hewison et al. 2019, Vogus & McClelland 2020, Ali &Terry 2017).

Reflective Activity: 1.4

Consider the definitions and theories outlined above.

Which theories and styles do you think apply well to your professional and practice context, and why?

Can you think of leaders you have worked with who apply these theories to their practice?

Write down the actions and behaviours that demonstrate the relevant approach and the impact on the service area or team or individuals.

1.4 SUMMARY

In this chapter we set out some of the leadership theories and considered how leadership is learnt. Understanding these theories will help you think about what kind of leader you want to be and what approach aligns with your personal and professional values. I hope the chapter has also ignited your interest further in being a leader in your profession. As American writer John Steinbeck put it on becoming a Nobel Laureate in 1962: "I am impelled, not to squeak like a grateful and apologetic mouse, but to roar like a lion out of pride in my profession."

This discussion may also offer some understanding and insight into how others demonstrate leadership; and hopefully, by reflecting on the theories outlined, it provides some further understanding of why leadership is important.

REFERENCES

Ali, S., & Terry, L. 2017. Exploring senior nurses' understanding of compassionate leadership in the community. *British Journal of Community Nursing*, 22(2), 77–87. https://doi.org/10.12968/bjcn.2017.22.2.77.

Avolio, B.J., & Gardner, W.L. 2005. Authentic leadership development: Getting to the root of positive forms of leadership. *Leadership Quarterly*, 16(3), 315–338.

Bennis, W., & Nanus, B. 1985. *Leaders: The strategies for taking charge*. New York: Harper & Row.

Bergman, J.Z., Rentsch, J.R., Small E.E. et al. 2012. The shared leadership process in decision-making teams. *Journal of Social Psychology*, 152(1), 17–42.

Burns, J.M. 1978. *Leadership*. New York: Harper & Row.

Clark, A., & Thompson, D. 2022. Nursing's leadership illusion? Time for more inclusive, credible and clearer conceptions of leadership and leaders. *Journal of Advanced Nursing*, 79(1), e1–e3.

Couarraze, S. et al. 2021. The major worldwide stress of healthcare professionals during the first wave of the COVID-19 pandemic: The international COVISTRESS survey. *PLoS ONE*, 16(10), e0257840. https://doi.org/10.1371/journal.pone.0257840.

de Zulueta, P.C. 2015. Developing compassionate leadership in health care: An integrative review. *Journal of Healthcare Leadership*, 8, 1–10. https://doi.org/10.2147/jhl.s93724.

Eicher-Catt, D. 2005. The myth of servant leadership: A feminist perspective. *Women and Language*, 28(1), 17–26.

Fiedler, F.E. 1967. *A theory of leadership effectiveness*. New York: McGraw-Hill.

Galton, F. 1869. *Hereditary genius*. New York: Appleton.

Greenfield, T.B. 1986. Leaders and school: Wilfulness and non-natural order in organizations. In Sergiovanni, T.J. & Corbally, J.E. (eds), *Leadership and organizational culture: New perspectives on administration theory and practice*, Chicago, IL: University of Chicago Press.

Greenleaf, R.K. 1977. *Servant leadership: A journey into the nature of legitimate power and greatness*. New York: Paulist Press.

Grossman, S., & Valiga, T.M. 2021. *The new leadership challenge: Creating the future of nursing*. 5th edn. Philadelphia, PA: F.A. Davis.

Handy, C. 1999. *Understanding organisations*. 3rd edn. London: Penguin.

Hanse, J.J., Harlin, U., Jarebrant, C. et al. 2016. The impact of servant leadership dimensions on leader–member exchange among health care professionals. *Journal of Nursing Management*, 24(2), 228–234. https://doi.org/10.1111/jonm.12304.

Henriksen, T.D., & Børgesen, K. 2016. Can good leadership be learned through business games? *Human Resource Development International*, 19(5), 388–405 https://doi.org/10.1080/13678868.2016.1203638.

Hersey, P., & Blanchard, K. 1988. *Management of organisational behaviour*. Englewood Cliffs, NJ: Prentice-Hall.

Hewison, A., Sawbridge, Y., & Tooley, L. 2019. Compassionate leadership in palliative and end-of-life care: A focus group study. *Leadership in Health Services*, 32(2), 264–279. https://doi.org/10.1108/lhs-09-2018-0044.

Hougaard, R., Carter, J., & Hobson, N. 2020. Compassionate leadership is necessary – but not sufficient. *Harvard Business Review*, 4 December. https://hbr.org/2020/12/compassionate-leadership-is-necessary-but-not-sufficient.

James, A.H., & Bennett, C.L. 2022. Power, politics and leadership. In Stanley, D., James, A.H., & Bennett, C.L. (eds), *Clinical leadership in nursing and healthcare*. 3rd edn. Hoboken: Wiley, pp. 385–402. https://doi.org/10.1002/9781119869375.ch18.

James, A.H., & Stanley, D. 2024. *Notes on … nursing leadership*. London: Wiley.

James, A.H., Dimond, R., Jones, A., Watkins, D., & Kelly, D. 2024a. Leading through the COVID 19 pandemic: Experiences of UK executive nurse directors. *Journal of Advanced Nursing*, 1–13. https://doi.org/10.1111/jan.16329.

James, A.H., Kelly, D., & Bennett, C.L. 2024b. Nursing tropes in turbulent times: Time to rethink nurse leadership? *Journal of Advanced Nursing*, 80, 8–10. https://doi.org/10.1111/jan.15766.

James, A.H., Watkins, D., & Carrier, J. 2022. Perceptions and experiences of leadership in undergraduate nurse education: A narrative inquiry. *Nurse Education Today*, 111, 105313. https://doi.org/10.1016/j.nedt.2022.105313.

Jones, L., & Bennett, C.L. 2018. *Leadership in health and social care: An introduction for emerging leaders*. 2nd edn. Banbury: Lantern.

Khan, Z.A., Nawaz, A., & Khan, I. 2016. Leadership theories and styles: A literature review. *Journal of Resources Development and Management*, 16, 1–7.

Kotter, J.P. 1990. *What leaders really do*. Boston, MA: Harvard Business School Press.

Leigh, A., & Maynard, M. 1995. *Leading your team: How to involve and inspire teams*. London: Nicholas Brealey.

Lett, M. 2002. The concept of clinical leadership. *Contemporary Nurse*, 12(1), 6–20.

Lowney, C. 2003. *Heroic leadership: Best practices from a 450-year-old company that changed the world*. Chicago, IL: Loyola.

Man, J. 2010. *The leadership secrets of Genghis Khan*. London: Bantam.

Mann, R.D. 1959. A review of the relationship between personality and performance in small groups. *Psychological Bulletin*, 56, 402–410.

Northouse, P.G. 2007. *Leadership: Theory and practice*. 4th edn. London: Sage.

Stanley, D. 2008. Congruent leadership: Values in action. *Journal of Nursing Management*, 16(5), 519–524. https://doi.org/10.1111/j.1365-2834.2008.00895.x.

Stanley, D. 2019. *Values-based leadership in healthcare: Congruent leadership explored*. London: Sage.

Stanley, D. 2022. Clinical leadership explored. In Stanley, D., Bennett, C.L., & James, A.H. (eds), *Clinical leadership in nursing and healthcare*. 3rd edn. Hoboken, NJ: Wiley, pp. 385–402. https://doi.org/10.1002/9781119869375.ch1.

Stanley, D., Bennett, C.L., & James, A. (eds). 2022. *Clinical leadership in nursing and healthcare*. 3rd edn. Hoboken, NJ: Wiley.

Steinbeck, J. 1962. The Nobel Prize: Banquet speech. https://www.nobelprize.org/prizes/literature/1962/steinbeck/speech/.

Stogdill, R.M. 1948. Personal factors associated with leadership: A survey of the literature. *Journal of Psychology*, 25, 35–71.

Tannenbaum, R., & Schmidt, W.H. 1958. How to choose a leadership pattern. *Harvard Business Review*, 36, 95–101.

Vogus, T.J., & McClelland, L.E. 2020. Actions, style and practices: How leaders ensure compassionate care delivery. *Leader*, 4(2), 48–52. https://doi.org/10.1136/leader-2020-000235.

Vroom, V.H., & Yetton, P. 1973. *Leadership and decision making*. Pittsburgh, PA: University of Pittsburgh Press.

West, M. 2021. *Compassionate leadership: Sustaining wisdom, humanity and presence in health and social*. Swirling Leaf Press.

Wong, C., & Cummings, G. 2009. Authentic leadership: A new theory for nursing or back to basics? *Journal of Health Organisations and Management*, 23(50), 522–538.

CHAPTER 2

LEADING DURING CHALLENGING TIMES
Lessons to take forward

Alison H. James

2.1 INTRODUCTION

This chapter will focus on the challenges of leading during difficult times. While we may feel that challenges present themselves frequently in our healthcare systems, there have been very challenging circumstances recently where effective leadership was essential to the delivery of healthcare and to the care of both staff and patients. It is important that any learning from these experiences is applied and captured for future planning, as I set out in Chapter 1, so that the different forms and experiences of learning are combined to form our learning and understanding of leading in a crisis. While healthcare crises have occurred across history – such as plagues, Cholera pandemics, influenza, and more recently outbreaks of Ebola – we have more recently seen a global impact during the COVID-19 pandemic caused by the rapid spread of the SARS-CoV-2 virus. The World Health Organization (WHO 2024) states that, since 2011, there have been more than 1,200 outbreaks of epidemic-prone diseases in 188 countries around the world.

The key role of the WHO is to coordinate and manage such events, maintaining and strengthening essential health services and systems globally or when countries and communities are in fragile, conflict-affected, and vulnerable circumstances. The WHO declared a *Public Health Emergency of International Concern* during COVID-19, the highest level of alarm, and it was clear that the vital role of leadership was essential from healthcare professionals in managing, containing, and providing healthcare services during the crisis. While there was a dearth of knowledge on healthcare crisis leadership pre-pandemic, what knowledge did exist focused on specific contexts and episodes, such as the earthquake in Christchurch, New Zealand or the Chilean miners' rescue (Zhuravsky 2015, Rashid et al. 2013).

Since 2020 much research has been completed and published to capture the lessons from the pandemic in the hope that all professions and public health leaders globally can build on the learning to inform future strategy and preparation for crises. Such evidence has provided suggestions for strategies of leading while also identifying the reality of healthcare systems in coping with such challenges. Strategic leadership within organisations is crucial at these times; however, individual leadership is also needed so that professionals can continue to lead the delivery of high standards of care, lead their teams in the challenges, and apply emotional intelligence to their practice.

An area of realisation and learning has also come from the portrayal of nurses and healthcare professionals during and since the pandemic. Certainly, for nurses, the imagery has varied, described by Bennett et al. (2020) and James et al. (2024b) as ranging from 'angelic tropes' to 'vexatious protestors', and other healthcare professionals have also struggled with such imagery. It could be said that these images, often portrayed via the media, do not help to encourage recruitment or ambition to lead for nursing and healthcare. However, this may also have the opposite effect, where challenges to our professional image encourage further determination to champion and vocalise the strengths of our professions and the vital need for leaders to build on the experience and take forward the lessons learnt.

DOI: 10.4324/9781003433354-3

Nurse leaders are highly skilled, safety-critical influencers and decision makers within healthcare, having considerable power and presence on the world stage for championing the profession (James et al. 2023, 2024a). Allied health professionals also hold highly valued skills, expertise, and experience to influence healthcare delivery with evidence and cohesion in a professional voice. While the pandemic was often traumatic and challenging for healthcare professionals, it is important that transparency and debate continue around some of the issues they were confronted with. For example, how effective was the 'command and control' styles of leadership which were often applied both by governments and health organisations to ensure quick decision making, action, and response? In our recent research exploring Executive Nurse Leaders and their leadership during the pandemic, we found that many who considered their usual style of leadership to be compassionate and empathetic applied a more autocratic approach due to the need for quick action (James et al. 2024a). Many told of the gratitude expressed by staff members to them for this clear and direct approach, which was highly valued during such uncertain and unpredictable times of crisis.

Reflective Activity: 2.1

Think about the adjectives associated with and used to describe your profession, whether it is nursing or any other allied health profession.

Do these adequately describe the potential and importance of the profession? What adjectives do you think should be used? Write these down.

Reflect on how important it is to champion and promote the positive roles of healthcare professions. How are the professions portrayed in the media and the nursing/healthcare press? Do these portrayals align with how you think they should?

2.2   LEADING IN A CRISIS AND BEYOND

A crisis can be defined as something immediate that poses a threat to the normal routine or functioning of everyday life. It is a time when often swift decisions must be made, actions taken, and the likelihood of change is high. James and Bennett (2020) suggest little change is needed to the knowledge and skills of leaders during a crisis; however what is imperative is the leaders' ability to adapt and attune their approach to respond to the stages of the crisis development. As mentioned in our previous study, Executive Nurse Leaders adapted their experience and knowledge of leadership styles to respond quickly and authoritatively, using one channel of clear communication (James et al. 2024a).

So, what makes a crisis different to challenging times? Currently, healthcare is experiencing challenging pressures following on from the crisis of COVID-19: not only because of the resources and demand the pandemic left in its wake, which in healthcare terms are yet to be determined as long-term effects of the virus emerge, but also because there are global macro challenges that also place demands on and barriers to provision of equitable healthcare, such as wars and other conflicts, financial constraints, and political instability. These and other challenges can impact our cultures of care and can directly impact the aspirations of providing high-quality effective and compassionate care. Even before the pandemic there are examples of where challenges to the values and beliefs of healthcare professions have had a negative impact and resulted in failures in care provision (Francis 2013).

In the UK and globally there has been a drive to recognise the importance of positive organisational cultures, especially during challenging times, and that these are heavily reliant on the leadership approach within the organisation. After all, organisations are made up of structures and systems; but the culture of an organisation is dependent on the people who lead and drive it forward. This can include chief executives and all through the levels of hierarchy and professions that exist within. In response to many of the serious case reviews and reports that have emerged from failures in care there is now recognition of the importance of aligning professional and organisational healthcare values with leadership throughout. These have also highlighted that nurturing positive and compassionate organisations has an impact on both patient outcomes and workforce wellbeing (West 2021).

Reflective Activity: 2.2 – Reframing and updating questions during a crisis or challenge

Consider the questions below, first from a team and organisational viewpoint and then from a personal level. Write down your answers and think about revisiting them regularly when you are facing challenging situations at work and reflect on previous answers as you develop your approach to leadership. You may find the answers change as you develop, and you may find it useful to revisit and reframe them according to your leadership progress. Often, when we reflect over time, it can be helpful to reset aims or realign to forgotten goals.

- What are the immediate desired outcomes (e.g. of the organisation or for yourself)?
- What are the longer-term desired outcomes?
- What are the current short-term, immediate aims?
- What are the longer-term aims?
- How will I communicate these effectively to my team and keep them supportive and engaged?
- What methods of communication have been effective previously for teamwork, and how can these be adapted for swift response and for longer-term response?
- What approach can I apply to influence the team and ensure all work to their strengths?
- What resources are needed to support the team to achieve the outcomes both in the immediate context and for the longer term?
- When will I review my approach to leading?
- When will I measure the effectiveness of my approach?
- How will I make myself available to others?
- How well are we meeting the organisation's values?
- How well are we meeting the values of our professions in the delivery of care?
- To what extent are my values anchored in my approach? Has this changed?
- To what extent will my values shape my approach to the application of ethically appropriate decisions and actions?
- How will I respond if my values are challenged?

Adapted from James and Bennett (2020).

We considered some of the values-based theories in Chapter 1 and explored why values are linked to leadership. Current values-based leadership theories emphasise the impact of positive relationships on patients and staff. For example, congruent leaders influence by making visible and acting according to their values and beliefs, aligning their vision for the organisation clearly with their values, demonstrated through their decision making and actions (Stanley et al. 2022). Compassionate leaders demonstrate values through empathy by being present, actively listening, being inquisitive about others and recognising pressures, and being curious about problems or mistakes, yet withholding blame and taking tangible actions to problem solve – that is, attending, understanding, empathising, and helping (West 2021). So, leaders are responsible for always influencing cultures, knowing their actions will be seen and role modelled in the hope this filters through the organisation. The importance of a values-based approach is accentuated in difficult and challenging times, where leaders set the tone of what is acceptable and professional behaviour and show continued expectations for high-quality practice through their own actions.

We suggest that leaders should self-question during times of crisis to enable a reframing of the context and consider immediate issues and demands (James & Bennett 2020). This approach has been adapted in *Reflective Activity 2.2* to include reflection and provide a longer-term view of ongoing challenges. Examples are included here for services; however, the same questions can be applied to individual outcomes and goals by changing *the* outcomes, *the* aims to *my* outcomes, *my* aims; and later questions are designed for personal leadership reflection. Remember, outcomes are the end result, product, state, or achievement. To know whether you have reached an outcome you will need to have a clear idea of how you might judge or measure it. For example, your personal desired outcome might be to develop your profile and experience as a professional by completing a Continuing Professional Development (CPD) programme even though, due to the challenges and pressure of work demands, time and funding availability have been reduced. Your measure would therefore be completion of the certificated programme. Similarly, in the context of work, the desired outcome may be to reduce patient waiting times for assessment, in which case the measure would be to establish how long waiting times are currently and set a time and number for reduction.

2.3   EFFECTS OF CHALLENGES AND CRISES

Before the COVID pandemic, it was recognised that those working in the health and social care domains in the UK were experiencing and reporting high levels of stress, depression, and anxiety (Health and Safety Executive 2021). Globally there has been concern for and discussion of the impact of *moral distress* and *moral injury* within the healthcare workforce and, during challenging times and crises, moral situations and conflicts tend to rise and can have profound and long-lasting effects on individuals and their intention to continue in their professions (Colville et al. 2019). While we deal with wellbeing and approaches for support in Chapter 7 of this book, here we consider some of the evidence and emerging thoughts on the impact on staff from crises and continual challenges, and how leaders may consider the impact on both themselves and on others.

While the terms 'moral distress' and 'moral injury' have many definitions in the literature, overall they can be considered as effects on the psychological, emotional, and physiological wellbeing of an individual when they experience moral dilemmas or moral conflict, or when actions are unaligned with ethical or moral values and principles (Morley et al. 2020, Watts et al. 2023). During the pandemic healthcare workers faced very difficult day-to-day challenges, and often they were the result of imposed directives, deemed necessary due to the unknown and uncertain nature of the virus and increased emotional burden from the nature of the professional work (James et al. 2024). Those working in health and social care faced ethical and moral dilemmas such as discharging potentially infected patients to family homes or care homes, risks to the professionals' own health and that of their families, and imposing visiting restrictions on families of critically ill patients. These situations were caused by *moral stressors* including working conditions, unavailable personal protective equipment (PPE), increased workloads, and unfamiliar clinical placements. For those who did have clinical and organisational decision-making responsibilities – such as executive-level staff, nurse leaders, and medical professionals – decisions lay in areas of patient care, staff/team care, and organisation/system care, placing extreme pressure on their moral and ethical balance.

Epstein et al. (2019) characterise morally distressing events as when individuals have low levels of influence on decision making, leading to feelings of lack of control and power, and possibly leading to what they feel is morally conflicting to their values. Feeling powerless and pressured can result in impressions of unimportance, and, if forced to act against their moral values, individuals can feel morally distressed and injured. While studies into moral distress and injury have been ongoing, and explored within many contexts outside of the pandemic, it is evident that the effect of moral distress can disrupt healthcare workers' physical and psychological health, wellbeing, and professional intentions (Watts et al. 2023).

Further causes of stress within the workforce include staffing levels and increased workloads, inflexible working schedules, discrimination and bullying, and levels of pay (West 2021). All these issues have been identified as increased stressors on staff in the UK and are reported globally. At some point this indicates a lack of effective high-level leadership. Of course, there are many excellent examples of organisational effectiveness, excellent patient care, and content workforces; however, it is important to recognise the different levels of leadership and influence within this very complex context of health and social care. For many leaders who are not in an organisational and hierarchical position, or who feel they are not, or feel unable to influence politics and or policy, taking a positive view may feel disingenuous and overwhelming. Here we need to refocus on values-based leadership and individual leadership, driven by self-awareness

---

Reflective Activity: 2.3

Based on our review of the literature and research on executive-level nurses during the COVID-19 pandemic, suggestions for support and enablers for positivity include the following:

- Identifying targeted support for inexperienced leaders (Hølge-Hazelton et al. 2021)
- Encouraging the development of supportive relationships between colleagues (Monroe et al. 2022), developing disaster policies, and increasing emergency resources (Freysteinson et al. 2021, He et al. 2022)
- Providing emotional health support and strategies for recovery for the workforce (Langan et al. 2022)
- Prioritising policies to support resilience and reduce burnout (Montgomery & Patrician 2022)
- Being flexible and adaptable during a crisis (Riggio & Newstead 2023)
- Encouraging support from peers, the flattening of hierarchy, and the removal of usual processes to allow and invite innovation (James et al. 2024).

Consider these suggestions. Do you agree with them; and what other suggestions do you think might support staff during crises and ongoing challenges?

and perspective. We also know that values-based approaches such as compassionate leadership can reduce staff burnout and affect staff wellbeing by reducing negative responses such as anxiety and incivility (Choi et al. 2016). Research exploring suffering has found that compassionate leaders ease staff suffering when confronted with challenging situations (Sánchez-Romero et al. 2022). So, by ensuring we act according to our professional values in how we approach others, how we listen carefully and with intent, how we respond, and how we analyse we can begin to address challenges with positive influence. As stated previously, those we lead will model behaviour based on what they experience and how that makes them feel (James et al. 2022).

2.4 MAINTAINING VALUES UNDER PRESSURE

While we may all agree that our professional values are central to our delivery of care and our ethical codes direct our decision making, the pressures of crises and challenging times place greater demands on us. Trying to maintain values when external and uncontrollable forces resist can be daunting and have consequences. Negative responses from those we hope to care for, and indeed colleagues, also have an impact. While facing anger and frustration, often taken out on those who are trying to help, it is important to revisit values and consider whether we are able to lead with compassion, care, courage, and empathy. Worline and Dutton (2017) suggest

---

Reflective Activity: 2.4

Here a student nurse describes the emotional impact and feelings on viewing the behaviour of others to the lead nurse. Reflecting on the challenges of relationships, the student also considers what this means for their future approach as a nurse leader.

> On a recent placement, there was a lot of staff on the wards, and it was quite cliquey … I thought, from an outside perspective, because I didn't know these nurses beforehand, the person who is in charge, being the leader, was very lovely and making what seemed to be sensible decisions, taking everyone into consideration. So, I thought it was unfair that other people were undermining her based on decisions that she had to do as her job. I hope I don't do that.
>
> If I am a leader eventually, I hope that I'm not talked about like that behind my back. It kind of made me a bit … I don't know, it's quite sad, if you're a leader … you can't also be friends with everyone … because to be a leader you have to be confident in your skills. Even now I don't think it's something I'm looking forward to but it hasn't built my confidence to see myself as a leader in the future.
>
> She was quite upset about it … she said it was part of being in charge … so she just accepted it and brushed it off. On the days when the nurse who was in the charge of the ward was on it was good, everyone was more confident in the decision being made that day. I suppose I felt that would be someone to look up to and if I was to, eventually, do that, that's the nurse that I'd want to be more like. If you don't have a role model to look to, you won't really know how nurses could lead and how they should do it.
>
> James (2020).

Consider times when you may have seen negative responses to another's leadership approach. Consider how you might respond to this if it challenges your professional values. Reflect on how this may be helpful for your practice as a leader.

that empathy and compassion trigger neural networks linked to altruism and social connection, and that what motivates healthcare professionals is the shared values that connect them. So, as Stanley and Stanley (2017) report from research and through the development of the congruent leadership theory, leaders who demonstrate values through actions in their real-world professional practice ensure visible connections between organisational, personal, and professional values. This reinforces accepted behaviours and legitimises compassionate approaches.

In my research of student nurses' experiences of leadership (James et al. 2022), students related how they had observed and experienced leadership and responses and reactions from other staff members. *Reflective activity 2.4* includes an excerpt from one student nurse's experience, demonstrating their thoughts on how the nurse leader managed the responses from her colleagues and how powerful the learning is from the emotions felt as an observer. What is clearly shown is how actions influence others, and how important positive role modelling is, even when it is challenging and perhaps easier to conform to pressure.

2.5 LEADING FOR SELF-CARE AND WELLBEING

While wellbeing is explored further in Chapter 7, here we consider actions and strategies from James and Bennett (2020), who set out a range of approaches as options, directed by need and context in our vastly different healthcare systems. What is common to all is our aim and determination to provide excellent care and lead through the challenges as they present themselves. Table 2.1 presents some of those approaches from the evidence that may be helpful during times of crises and day-to-day trials.

Thompson and Kusy (2021) recommend the space and time for sharing experiences and personal stories; and emotional expression can make a significant contribution not only to the individual, in being listened to, but also to those who listen and read the stories. This aspect of relating experience can add to the development of knowledge, evidence, and thinking, and lead to the development of new approaches and learning (James et al. 2022). While they may change and adapt as people rely on recall of events, stories can be a powerful way to connect people and identify parallels in experience, which allow associations and relationship building

Table 2.1 Leadership strategies for wellbeing

Strategy	Source
Provide opportunities for sharing stories, emotions, and reflection in a safe place to avoid suppression and fear	Thompson and Kusy (2021), James et al. (2022)
Mindfulness techniques can decrease emotional tiredness; enabling staff to access these can support their wellbeing	Klatt et al. (2017)
Mentorship and buddying can support new staff and staff development	King's Fund (2021)
Be a visible leader to staff and senior leadership, representing and advocating for staff wellbeing as a priority	Markey et al. (2020)
Role model demonstrating a compassionate, cohesive, and positive approach, encouraging a positive culture	King's Fund (2021)
Provide clear and effective communication to all staff, especially when policy or directives change rapidly, ensuring time for questions, active listening, and responding to concerns	Rosa et al. (2020), Lasater et al. (2021), James et al. (2024b)

Adapted from James and Bennett (2020).

and reduce feelings of isolation, especially in times of adversity or crisis. It may also be helpful to explore others' thoughts on facing challenging situations; and a simple line of thought can be impactful, cause us to pause and consider, and help us move forward. For example, think of this line from Leonard Cohen, a poet and song writer who managed to capture a moment of difficulty and yet make it positive: "There is a crack in everything. That's how the light gets in" (2015, p. 366).

We explore the useful nature of journaling and storytelling further in Chapter 10 as these can be powerful methods of self-development and personal leadership maturity.

2.6   POSITIVE DISRUPTIVE LEADERSHIP

While the evidence tells us that compassionate and values-based leadership is effective, learning from the COVID crisis also allows some further consideration of *positive disruptive leadership* approaches. Disruptive leaders are those who often seek solutions and ways to improve productivity, improve end outcomes, and ensure systems and processes function well. They aren't afraid to challenge conventional wisdom. In healthcare, risk can be a tricky concept as we are dealing with human life, not commercial products, and this makes disruptive leadership less attractive to some. We base our decisions on evidence rather than experimenting with new ideas – and of course this is essential for safe patient care, and ethically correct. So how can we use lessons of disruptive leadership from business and management to make positive innovation without increasing risk for our patients? How can we challenge and question top-down policy and innovate for improvement in patient care and for staff conditions at work? If we agree that leaders can positively affect innovation, then as long as values and ethical codes are kept focused, the results can be positive.

Leading in unfamiliar and high-stress situations requires order, and some degree of process, so that insight, analysis, and later scrutiny can occur. Our research exploring Executive Nurses' experiences of leadership during the pandemic found that this was a continuous thread in the data (James et al. 2024a). While policies were in place, reports of innovation and creative approaches, alongside the removal of 'usual procedures' that would usually slow processes down, were positive aspects for many. There was also recognition that, while thinking on their feet was necessary, the research participants were fully aware that when the crisis had passed and normal times returned, detail and scrutiny of decision making were expected. While many were grasping innovation and taking some risks, their professionalism and experience as leaders were central to guiding their decisions in a very uncertain and highly stressful time (James et al. 2024a). What also became clear was that, following the crisis, often some of the best innovations were lost, practice reverted to pre-crisis, and red tape restrictions returned.

Many of the most effective leaders in business and industry expect crises rather than consider their improbability. Preparation for the worst-case scenario is part of sound strategic planning, which is why there are plans for disaster management and serious events within many governmental policies. However, anticipating crisis often requires innovation, and innovation often requires resources. This is perhaps where some of our health organisations are disadvantaged and weakened in a crisis as resources are often finite and focused on the most immediate need and routine innovation, rather than investment in future and pre-emptive innovation. As witnessed in the pandemic, many organisations responded with rapid reorganisation and effective innovation under extreme stress, most likely using policies which had been established and agreed on prior to the event. What we know about crises is that there is always a 'curve ball', and there will be a need for a new way of thinking, a creative initiative alongside a fear for the unknown.

On an individual level, depending on the area, health and social care workers will have strategies and policies, preparation, and training for managing crises and serious events locally. Keeping to these policies in professions that deal with human life is of course important and reduces the risk of harm to the people we care for. However, we may not be prepared for the responsibilities and challenges we face when confronted by a disaster on the level of the pandemic. Having some pre-emptive approaches in preparation for leadership can be challenging, depending on experience, knowledge, and confidence. However, as you gain experience in your profession, this may also give you a glimpse of possibilities and potential for innovation. Being open to innovative ideas, developing a wider perspective outside of the local situation, being open to working across professions and boundaries, and having the courage to speak up can be defined as 'positive disruptive leadership'.

Disruptive leadership in healthcare requires a global perspective, a multidisciplinary focus, experience and knowledge of the evidence, and an empathetic and compassionate perspective. Change is only implemented when evidenced as a need, and leads to an increase in value – whether that is through improving patient care, improving care pathways, unblocking bottlenecks and delays, or improving staff morale, among others.

Reflective Activity: 2.5

Disruptive leaders see the bigger picture, think 'outside the box', and are curious and seeking solutions while remaining empathetic and compassionate.

Examples of disruptive leadership are evident in some of the initiatives that occurred during the pandemic, when decisions had to be made to work differently, move services and professionals into different areas and specialities, and develop field hospitals and vaccination programmes. Despite the restrictions imposed, such as banning relatives from visiting and mandatory masking for safety, many innovative approaches were created and implemented to find solutions. Many healthcare leaders made concerted efforts to be visible to staff, to actively listen, and to set up different and regular forms of communications (such as Zoom calls) to push through initiatives to improve conditions for staff and patients where usual rules and regulations may have been prohibited.

Reflect on the positive and potentially risky aspects of disruptive leadership, especially in terms of you as an individual practitioner and to wider healthcare.

Reflect on any examples you can think of where a wider perspective has supported and effected change in practice. What were the risks and what were the benefits to patient care?

Qualities associated with positive disruptive leaders include:

- Fearlessness to ensure high standards, applying evidence in decision making, and speaking up.
- Being decisive and inspiring confidence – clarity of vision and excellent communication of the vision and how it will be achieved.
- Being adaptable and flexible – opportunities are seen in failures and challenges, learning from events that others may see as in the past and best forgotten.
- Life-long and continual learning – championing learning and encouraging it in others; seeking inspiration outside of the usual areas and seeking support from role models through coaching and training.

- Understanding others and seeking to understand their uncertainty and concerns; maintaining focus and being comfortable with uncertainty.

- Putting patients at the centre; problem solving and constantly seeking solutions and innovative ways to ensure high standards of care.

- Challenging and sometimes breaking with convention; questioning and scrutinising for clarity.

The qualities above, when combined with elements of values-based leadership, can be powerful for innovative improvements in patient care. However there are models of leadership that could have the opposite effect when combined with this approach, with risks of narcissism and autocracy. So, while disruptive leadership does not suit everyone, it can be effective in applying learning and focusing for improvement.

2.7   CONCLUSION

This chapter has explored the challenges of leading during a crisis and in difficult times. We have considered impacts and positive and negative influences, and some of the evidence that allows learning and planning for the future. For personal leadership the importance of taking time to reflect, to express emotions of experience and acknowledge the impact of emotional experiences can encourage deeper critical thinking and foster emotional intelligence. We also considered the possibilities for positive disruptive leadership, its usefulness in learning from challenges and how it can be helpful if applied with a values-based approach. Further approaches to wellbeing are presented in Chapter 7, which we hope further support these aspects of your leadership growth; and we also explore techniques such as journaling and storytelling in Part 2 of this book.

REFERENCES

Bennett, C., James, A.H., & Kelly, D. 2020. Beyond tropes: Towards a new image of nursing in the wake of COVID-19. *Journal of Clinical Nursing*, 29(15–15), 2753–2755. http://dx.doi.org/10.1111/jocn.15346.

Choi, H.J., Lee, S., No, S., & Kim, E.I. 2016. Effects of compassion on employees' self-regulation. *Social Behavior and Personality: An International Journal*, 44 (7), 1173–1190.

Cohen, L. 2015. Anthem. In Berger, J. (ed.), *Leonard Cohen on Leonard Cohen: Interviews and encounters. Musicians in their own words*. Chicago Review Press.

Colville, G., Dawson, D., Rabinthiran, S., Chaudry-Daley, Z., & Perkins-Porras, L. 2019. A survey of moral distress in staff working in intensive care in the UK. *Journal of the Intensive Care Society*, 20, 196–203. https://doi.org/10.1177/1751143718787753.

Epstein, E.G., Whitehead, P.B., Prompahakul, C., Thacker, L.R., & Hamric, A.B. 2019. Enhancing understanding of moral distress: The measure of moral distress for health care professionals. *AJOB Empirical Bioethics*, 10, 113–124. https://doi.org/10.1080/23294 515.2019.158600.

Francis, R. 2013. *Report of the Mid Staffordshire NHS Foundation Trust Public Inquiry*. Norwich: The Stationery Office.

Freysteinson, W.M., Celia, T., Gilroy, H., & Gonzalez K. 2021. The experience of nursing leadership in a crisis: A hermeneutic phenomenological study. *Journal of Nursing Management*, 29(6), 1535–1543.

He, L.X., Ren, H.F., Chen F.J., et al. 2022. Perspectives of nursing directors on emergency nurse deployment during the pandemic of COVID-19: A nationwide cross-sectional survey in mainland China. *Journal of Nursing Management*, 30(5), 1147–1156.

Health and Safety Executive. 2021. *Health and Safety Executive annual report and accounts 2020/21*. https://assets.publishing.service.gov.uk/media/614339a2e90e0704352cbc06/hse-annual-report-and-accounts-2020-2021.pdf.

Hølge-Hazelton, B., Kjerholt M., Rosted E., et al. 2021. Health professional frontline leaders' experiences during the COVID-19 pandemic: A cross-sectional study. *Journal of Healthcare Leadership*, 13, 7–18.

James, A.H. 2020. *Perceptions and experiences of leadership: A narrative inquiry of leadership in undergraduate nurse education.* Doctoral thesis, Cardiff University. https://orca.cardiff.ac.uk/id/eprint/140444.

James, A.H., & Bennett, C. 2020. Effective nurse leadership in times of crisis. *Nursing Management,* 27(4), 32–40. https://doi.org/10.7748/nm.2020.e1936.

James, A.H., Dimond, R., Jones, A., Watkins, D., & Kelly, D. 2024a. Leading through the COVID 19 pandemic: Experiences of UK executive nurse directors. *Journal of Advanced Nursing,* 1–13. https://doi.org/10.1111/jan.16329.

James, A.H., Kelly, D., & Bennett, C. L. 2024b. Nursing tropes in turbulent times: Time to rethink nurse leadership? *Journal of Advanced Nursing,* 80, 810. https://doi.org/10.1111/jan.15766.

James, A.H., Watkins, D., & Carrier, J. 2022. Perceptions and experiences of leadership in undergraduate nurse education: A narrative inquiry. *Nurse Education Today,* 111, 105313. https://doi.org/10.1016/j.nedt.2022.105313.

King's Fund. 2021. Compassionate and inclusive leadership. https://www.kingsfund.org.uk/insight-and-analysis/projects/compassionate-and-inclusive-leadership.

Klatt, M.D., Weinhold, K., Taylor, C.A., Zuber, K., & Sieck, C.J. 2017. A pragmatic introduction of mindfulness in a continuing education setting: Exploring personal experience, bridging to professional practice. *Explore,* 13(5), 327–332. https://doi.org/10.1016/j.explore.2017.06.003.

Lasater, K.B., Aiken, L.H., Sloane, D.M., et al. 2021. Chronic hospital nurse understaffing meets COVID-19: An observational study. *BMJ Quality & Safety,* 30, 639–647. https://doi.org/10.1136/bmjqs-2020-011512.

Markey, K., Ventura, C.A.A., O'Donnell C., & Doody, O. 2020. Cultivating ethical leadership in the recovery of COVID-19. *Journal of Nursing Management,* 29(2), 351–355.

Montgomery, A.P., & Patrician, P.A. 2022. Work environment, resilience, burnout, intent to leave during COVID pandemic among nurse leaders: A cross-sectional study. *Journal of Nursing Management,* 30(8), 4015–4023.

Morley, G., Bradbury-Jones, C., & Ives, J. 2020. What is 'moral distress' in nursing? A feminist empirical bioethics study. *Nursing Ethics,* 27, 1297–1314. https://doi.org/10.1177/0969733019874492.

Rashid, F., Edmondson, A.C., & Leonard, H.B. 2013. Leadership lessons from the Chilean mine rescue. *Harvard Business Review,* 91(7–8), 113–119, 134. PMID: 24730174.

Riggio, R.E., & Newstead, T. 2023. Crisis leadership. *Annual Review of Organizational Psychology and Organizational Behavior,* 10, 201–224.

Rosa, W.E., Schlak, A.E., & Rushton, C.H. 2020. A blueprint for leadership during COVID-19. *Nursing Management,* 51(8), 28–34. https://doi.org/10.1097/01.NUMA.0000688940.29231.6f.

Sánchez-Romero, S., Ruiz-Fernández, M.D., Fernández-Medina, I.M., et al. 2022. Experiences of suffering among nursing professionals during the COVID-19 pandemic: A descriptive qualitative study. *Applied Nursing Research,* 66, 151603.

Stanley, D. & Stanley, K. 2017. Clinical leadership and nursing explored: A literature search. *Journal of Clinical Nursing,* 27: 1730–1743.

Stanley, D., Bennett, C.L., & James, A.H. (eds). 2022 *Clinical leadership in nursing and healthcare.* Hoboken, NJ: Wiley.

Thomson, R., & Kusy, M. 2021. Has the COVID pandemic strengthened or weakened health care teams? A field guide to health workforce best practices. *Nursing Administration Quarterly,* 45(2), 135–141.

Watts, T., Sydor, A., Whybrow, D. et al. 2023. Registered nurses' and nursing students' perspectives on moral distress and its effects: A mixed-methods systematic review and thematic synthesis. *Nursing Open,* 10, 6014–6032. doi:10.1002/nop2.1913.

West, M. 2021. *Compassionate leadership: Sustaining wisdom, humanity and presence in health and social.* Swirling Leaf Press.

World Health Organization. 2024. Health emergencies. https://www.who.int/our-work/health-emergencies [Accessed 5 June 2024].

Worline, M., & Dutton, J.E. 2017. *Awakening compassion at work: The quiet power.* Oakland, CA: Berrett-Koehler.

Zhuravsky, L. 2015. Crisis leadership in an acute clinical setting: Christchurch hospital, New Zealand ICU experience following the February 2011 earthquake. *Prehospital and Disaster Medicine,* 30(2), 131–136. doi:10.1017/S1049023X15000059.

CHAPTER 3

POWER, POLITICS, AND SOCIAL JUSTICE
Developing your voice and being heard

Alison H. James

3.1 INTRODUCTION

In this chapter we begin to explore the significance of power, politics, and social justice to leadership and some of the challenges of influencing, both locally and in wider contexts. Developing a confident *voice* is part of developing your leadership, and you can of course choose where and how to do this. It may be that you want to nurture and mentor others locally, or you may feel your profession needs a louder voice, a greater say in the wider healthcare debate and decision making. That is of course for the individual to decide; however, whatever level you choose to influence, it is important to understand and acknowledge that power and politics are central directors, influencing the resources we have to deliver patient care and support staff. I would also suggest that all healthcare professionals should be engaged and aware of the inter-relationship of power and politics and their influence on the outcomes for patients, the equity of resource allocation, and how decisions are made as they are delivering these for patients.

3.2 UNDERSTANDING POWER

From an early age, we begin to form our views on power through contact and interaction with adults and, perhaps even more now, through contact with cultural products such as the internet and television (Hilty et al. 2023, Howard & Gill 2000). Social experiences, whether face to face or more remotely through social media, will involve various balances of power, and there will always be differences in those levels of power. Politics is also considered alongside power in this chapter; and, while leadership is integral to politics, you may wonder why it is included in this self-leadership context. When considering the definition of politics, there are two contexts: politics that determines the governance of a country or state; and what we sometimes call *soft* or *small politics*, which concerns the relationships in organisations, groups or cultures that determine levels of power balance. Both contexts involve levels and types of power; and in both contexts they can be highly influential on our workplace cultures, on our experience of leadership in organisations, and in the wider delivery and allocation of health and care.

We may feel that we are in control of the conversation when interacting with social media, naively thinking there are no further agendas to some of these interactions. For example, concerns have been raised and debate continues as to whether social media platforms should be regulated; and instances of alleged interference in elections and referendums have raised concerns of external power directing internal decisions on wider scales (Ghosh 2021). These concerns thus recognise abuse of power at both the individual level and on a wider scale. As with many concepts, a firm and agreed definition of power is challenging and can depend on the relevant context. However, in terms of leadership, power in itself is not good or bad, not wholly positive or negative. However, overall it is *influencing*, evokes a *response*, and has an *effect*. What these are depends on how it is applied and what the purpose is. Marquis and Houston (2012) state that power is needed in all leadership, and that how it is applied and the effect it has depend on the intention and aim of the leader. The authors also agreed that there are different types of power, including self-power, which means having power over your own life, applying maturity, confidence and being secure to

DOI: 10.4324/9781003433354-4

develop personal strength. This self-power is an aspect of overall personal leadership and is linked to emotional intelligence (explored further in Chapter 5) and wellbeing (Chapter 7).

Power and politics are also present in wider contexts, globally and geographically; they will have shaped our society and culture historically as well as the relationship between governments and health and social care provision. So, if we consider how resources are distributed and healthcare systems function internationally, there will be discrepancies and differences. The World Health Organization (WHO) Commission on the Social Determinants of Health (CSDH 2008, p. 1) states that health inequalities exist due to "a toxic combination of poor social policies and programmes, unfair economic arrangements and bad politics". Developing a wider awareness of these issues is therefore important to cultivate a broader appreciation of the impact of power and policies on the wellbeing of health and social care delivery globally.

The balance of power between professions and professionals can influence how effectively a team works together. This can be determined by who leads the team and what value is placed and communicated to each member of that team (James & Bennett 2023). In the context of healthcare, professional leadership suggests that power influences positive aspects and encourages effective relationships. However, we must also acknowledge the concept of powerlessness, or the feeling of having no influence. Sometimes, we may perceive we have no power; this can be a common aspect of working in large organisations, where we feel disconnected from the decision making and direction of policies we are told to conform to (James & Bennett 2023). However, perceptions can change and, as leaders, if we wish to make change, whether in situations or in terms of perceptions, with support and by seeking opportunities, engaging with others, and gaining knowledge in the power structures involved change can be achieved (see Chapter 6 for more thoughts on change).

Power can also be abused and enable negative outcomes for individuals and organisations; and this can be done with deliberate consciousness or indeed by unintended actions. In healthcare there are examples of professional abuse of power that may or may not be deliberate, and this is often witnessed in teams and professions through cultures of behaviours and rituals that are allowed to continue rather than questioned. Indeed, in nursing, issues of bullying and incivility are ongoing topics of concern, especially for student nurses who report incidents of challenging behaviour and misuse of power relationships on the part of those who are supposed to be their role models (Darbyshire et al. 2019, James 2023). For the nursing profession, where shortages of both qualified and student nurses is a global issue, the message of zero tolerance of negative behaviour must be communicated clearly when required to ensure that behaviour and use of power reflect professional values when applied to patients and colleagues.

Being aware of the types of power and how they are used can be helpful to leaders in identifying and challenging misuse where necessary. Yoder-Wise (2015) provides some examples of types of power:

- Resource power – the ability to allocate resources and budgets, development and promotion opportunities, rewards and punishment through withholding
- Information power – possessing information or knowledge, and having the ability to share or withhold it
- Expert power – developing knowledge and experience that hold value in certain situations
- Coercive power – applying power to invoke threat or fear
- Charismatic power – the ability to form connections and relationships with those in positions of authority
- Legitimate power – holding a titled position that suggests authority over others
- Reward power – having the ability to award or reward by methods others value.

> **Reflective Activity: 3.1**
>
> Firstly consider: How would you define power?
>
> Write down your thoughts and think about your experiences of power.
>
> Thinking about the types of power listed above, write down your experiences of these being held or used. Consider how they were applied.
>
> How would you apply these types of power as a leader?
>
> Secondly, consider the following quote from the novel *The Cat's Table* by Michael Ondaatje (2012, p. 103). What type of power is being described here, and how does this relate to culture and organisations? Write down your thoughts.
>
> That was a small lesson I learned on the journey. What is interesting and important happens mostly in secret, in places where there is no power. Nothing much of lasting value ever happens at the head of the table, held together by familiar rhetoric. Those who already have power continue to glide along the familiar rut they have made for themselves.

3.3   SOCIAL JUSTICE AND CRITICAL SOCIAL THEORY

Critical social theory is centred on social justice, empowerment and the relationships between knowledge, ideology and power within learning and experience. Healthcare professions focus on delivering care that aims to be fair, just and equal; therefore, social justice is core to this concept and core to our professional service to society. The COVID-19 pandemic provides examples of where countries and governments demonstrated their fundamental effectiveness in applying frameworks of justice in preventing premature mortality and reducing the risk of spread (Ruger 2020); and demonstrations of ethical leadership were tangible through actions and policies which were grounded in good morals and evidenced honesty, integrity and transparency. There were examples of social justice from leaders who acted with their ethical values clearly visible through regard for all people and populations. Some of the countries with the most effective responses to the pandemic included South Korea, Germany, Finland and New Zealand, where leaders recognised the that shared values and responsibilities were needed for the population, and communicating these was effectively clear (Ruger 2020).

We have argued that healthcare cannot be detached from social, economic and political influences (James et al. 2021). In developing a personal and professional approach to leadership, social consciousness and awareness are required if we are to serve our communities and attend to the diverse populations and wider issues that impact healthcare globally (James & Bennett 2023). Also intertwined with social justice are professional ethics and moral principles, so its relevance is bound to our professional obligations and requirements. However, this presents us with challenges; examples would be the availability and distribution of vaccines, provision and access to healthcare in countries in conflict, and the use of misinformation in healthcare science. All place obligations on healthcare professionals to provide equal care and enable access to care; however, power and politics mean this may not always be possible.

There are also concerns about healthcare professionals' knowledge and awareness of what social justice is, and whether it is given due prominence by our regulators and through our education programmes (Valderama-Wallace & Apesoa-Varano 2019, Habibzadeh et al. 2021). While students learn about professional ethics and values, they are perhaps less aware of the wider implications and the wider influencing factors that keep inequities in healthcare present in some countries. The COVID-19 pandemic has increased global awareness of local and community roles in both protecting and promoting health; however, as mentioned previously, the learning and initiatives from this time risks being lost (James et al. 2024, Mannion et al. 2023). Indeed, some consider the focus on local initiatives for improving health and supporting local empowerment of communities to be promoting an 'inward gaze' rather than focusing on the wider political and social transformative policies that could address a wider approach to really tackling health and social inequities (Popay et al. 2020). Empowerment and emancipation are considered further in Chapter 4 exploring the role, and arguably the responsibility, of health leaders to be actively concerned with these concepts within the spectrum of power and the complexities of healthcare systems.

Critical social theory is a way of exploring the oppressive use of power in societies (Giroux 1983), and is a collection of theories rather than a distinct concept. This approach seeks to make sense of a social order to invoke transformation and shifts in power, so it can be influential in the context of challenges and for leadership. Critical social theory focuses on the challenges of *false consciousness* of members of society. Through reframing the situation, explaining and making clear the situation in a different way, individuals may think of things differently, which would be explained as *enlightening the oppressed*. Once enlightened, a group may decide to take action and become empowered, achieving emancipation and freedom from the constraints that overpowered them. A hypothetical example in healthcare is presented in Box 3.1.

Box 3.1 Hypothetical example of enlightening the oppressed

Imagine that nursing and allied healthcare professions have been historically based on concepts of altruism and unquestioning obedience to the medical profession and governing political parties. (Remember this is hypothetical!)

Some nurses and allied health professionals begin to question this subservient role and begin to realise that they could provide better care for their patients and extend their role and influence by changing and moving from subservient roles to being more autonomous professionals. However, these enlightened professionals realise that not every nurse and allied health professional wishes to acknowledge or be conscious of their subservient and oppressed position.

To change this state, the enlightened professionals begin to educate others in the potential of being less oppressed by offering the benefits of influencing care and evidence, and also through better social standing and influence, better work conditions, better pay, and so on. Now imagine that this group of professionals are the largest by number and hold power in their ability to mobilise and change their oppressed position, improving the care they provide, the services they run as well as their own personal standing and reward.

In the context of healthcare and social justice, the approach in Box 3.1 can be impactful and help make change where disparities exist. To achieve this, Fay (1987) advocates the three-stage process of enlightenment, empowerment and emancipation, applying the following theories:

- False consciousness – where a group or society has adopted the views, values and beliefs of a more dominant influence, and becomes oppressed.
- Crisis theory – the examination of dissatisfaction in a group and how this can dissipate group cohesion.

- Education theory – how enlightenment is best achieved.
- Transformative action – identification of what requires changing to achieve resolution in a crisis and enable a plan of action.

While healthcare professionals are clear in their role as advocates for patient care, and most are experienced in advocating locally for their patients, the role is not always embraced on a wider political scale. Wider political influence may seem beyond the scope and ability of many; and, of the professions, nursing is often not valued as a political and powerful force to engage with on wider healthcare issues. The pandemic highlighted this across all professions; and, while valued in the delivery of care, nurses were not influential when it came to wider decision making at the higher levels of political concern (Bennett et al. 2020).

As healthcare leaders, if we are to have influence and engage in the decisions that are directed at the macro level and influence what we then deliver at the meso and micro levels, there is a requirement to gain full knowledge and evidence, to be able to identify priorities, and to understand the wider political agendas and population needs (Yoder-Wise 2015, James & Bennett 2023). Equally, to do this, we must develop confidence in personal leadership and excellence in communication skills, negotiation skills and collaborative working, alongside a level of political astuteness to match those around the table. What is important here is to consider in this context the overall personal philosophy of leadership. We discussed the importance of ethical codes and values in earlier chapters, so keeping your values central to the approach is essential when considering aspects of power and any political position of influence.

3.4   BECOMING POLITICALLY AWARE AND ACTIVE

Being a politically active healthcare professional means being actively engaged with the debate, standing up for your profession and values, and taking action to gain a voice and be heard. This can be done on a range of levels depending on what you want to achieve, how confident you are and how passionate you are in engaging in the wider issues. Contexts for engagement range from your clinical field to the wider organisation, a local area or country, and even the global arena. Without being radical or extreme, which polarises beliefs and reduces knowledgeable debate, there are many ways begin to develop your *voice*, represent your profession and lead for change. The following are a few examples:

- Join committees or professional associations to increase your network and contact list. Explore international areas of interest and associations to join to widen your opportunities for networking and to learn from the international communities of professions.
- Identify what is possible within your area (this could begin locally in the clinical area and expand to the community and wider) and take action to make change if needed to improve any aspect of care delivery.
- Engage with professional issues; take part in discussions and debates to have your voice heard.
- Contribute to publications and articles in your professional journals. Some people create blogs and invite colleagues for discussion in podcasts. Find out if there are accessible areas or consider creating them yourself.
- Be interested in and informed about what is happening in the wider health policy agenda, both within your profession and that of other professions. Read and access reliable sources of information.
- Look for accessible conferences to attend and contribute to and join in the debates.

3.5 INFLUENCING STYLES

If we accept that leadership involves influencing, and that power is related to influencing, then understanding how they are linked and how you can develop these for positive impact should be an element of your self-development journey. Applying influence well will depend on your capacity to demonstrate and engage effective interpersonal skills and emotional intelligence. Encouraging others to change behaviours and attitudes lies with the leader's ability to manage power and develop strategies to empower others (James & Bennett 2023). Use of the strategies chosen will depend on your preferred leadership style, your relationship with others and the openness of others to be influenced. It may be that you will need to alter your approach if it is not working, and you may need to adopt a different approach depending on the people and circumstances you are seeking to influence. Being flexible and open to this are therefore important skills for leaders to possess. Table 3.1 outlines some influencing styles you may want to apply and consider using in practice.

Power then is only potential until the individual masters the ability to influence others (Bragg 1996). To work towards increasing your influence, there are ways of developing aspects of your skill set. These include:

- **Gaining knowledge and skills.** A sound and wide knowledge base can be long-lasting and influence areas outside of your speciality. However, gaining specialised knowledge is also effective and can establish your position as someone who holds a high level of knowledge in an area, thereby establishing your own position.
- **Establishing legitimacy.** Demonstrating your values and beliefs through actions that align to your profession and to your organisation's ethos. Articulating your values and being consistent can convince others of your aims and vision.
- **Always making the effort.** Making an effort within your organisation will establish your dedication and commitment and be visible to others. Contributing to and being involved in your organisation's functions and aims will furnish you with a reputation

Table 3.1 Influencing styles

Style	Summary
Assertive persuasion	A logical and calculated approach that aims to influence by reason and force of argument and counterargument. Using facts and evidence to support your argument will of course help with this approach.
Reward and punishment	Influencing others by use of incentives or disincentives to control their behaviours. Power can be asserted using direct and forceful approaches, or through the imbalance of power and status or hierarchy.
Participation and trust	Active listening and engagement are part of this approach. Being open and honest can influence others to also be transparent and voice their thoughts, and also feel valued.
Common values	If the leader demonstrates their values through their actions, they will appeal to those who share those values, and appeals are made to their emotions, evoking enthusiasm and excitement for change.
Common vision	As with common values, this approach appeals to those who share the vision described by the leader. Members of a group will realise their potential as a group and feel valued as part of that vision if this is communicated clearly by a leader. Finding a common aim and goal encourages people to work as a team.

Adapted from James and Bennett (2023).

as a valued member of staff and someone who has enthusiasm to make something successful.

- **Being personable.** Being pleasant, responsive and helpful may seem obvious, but these attributes are viewed positively and can establish you as someone who is approachable, trustworthy and agreeable. Unnecessary conflicts, discussing others negatively to some or being agreeable to some and not all can give the opposite impression, and levels of trust will soon diminish.

- **Gaining a reputation for responding and acting.** Being on time for meetings, being fully prepared, taking action on commitments and actively listening to everyone in the room can all be important in establishing your reputation as reliable, focused and interested in others' contributions.

Reflective Activity: 3.2

Think about at least one person you consider holds a degree of power at work. How are you aware of this power? This could be through behaviours or actions. Write these behaviours or actions down.

Now consider how you view this person's leadership. Do their actions reflect the type of leader they are? Do you think they are aware of their use of power and how this influences others?

Do you think you have power in your area of work? If so, what sort of power is it? Do you think others are aware of this?

How can power impact patient care? Reflect on this and write down positive and negative influences of power on patients and patient safety.

3.6 SUMMARY

In this chapter we have explored the significance of power, politics and social justice to leadership and some of the challenges of influencing, both locally and in wider contexts. It may also have made you consider how health professions, health professionals and organisations use power and are subjected to power, and the role of politics within those areas. It is important for your personal leadership development to be aware of the power dynamics at play within work contexts and how this can impact your practice and your leadership approach. Ultimately, the use of power in this context also affects patient care. It is therefore worth considering further what this concept means, and how it can be applied to effect positive change and improvement as well as support how you develop relationships with individuals and teams to gain influence for the benefit of your career, your profession and your patients.

REFERENCES

Bennett, C., James, A., & Kelly, D. 2020. Beyond tropes: Towards a new image of nursing in the wake of COVID-19. *Journal of Clinical Nursing*, 29(15–16), 2753–2755. http://dx.doi.org/10.1111/jocn.15346.

Bragg, M. 1996. *Reinventing influence: How to get things done in a world without authority*. London: Pitman.

CSDH. 2008. *Closing the gap in a generation: Health equity through action on the social determinants of health. Final Report of the Commission on Social Determinants of Health*. Geneva: World Health Organization.

Darbyshire, P., Thompson, D.R., & Watson, R. 2019. Nursing's future? Eat young. Spit out. Repeat. Endlessly. *Journal of Nursing Management*, 27(7),1337–1340. https://doi.org/10.1111/jonm.12781.

Fay, B. 1987. *Critical social science: Liberation and its limits*. Ithaca, NY: Cornell University Press.

Ghosh, D. 2021. Are we entering a new era of social media regulation? *Harvard Business Review*, 14 January. https://hbr.org/2021/01/are-we-entering-a-new-era-of-social-media-regulation.

Giroux, H.A. 1983. *Theory and resistance in education*. London: Heinemann.

Habibzadeh, H., Jasemi, M., & Hosseinzadegan, F. (2021). Social justice in health system; a neglected component of academic nursing education: A qualitative study. *BMC Nursing*, 20, Art 16. https://doi.org/10.1186/s12912-021-00534-1.

Hilty, D.M., et al. 2023. A scoping review of social media in child, adolescents and young adults: Research findings in depression, anxiety and other clinical challenges. *BJPsych Open*, 9(5), e152. https://doi.org/10.1192/bjo.2023.523.

Howard, S., & Gill, J. 2000. The pebble in the pond: Children's construction of power, politics and democratic citizenship. *Cambridge Journal of Education*, 30(3), 357–358.

James, A.H. 2023. Valuing the emotions of leadership learning in nurse education. *Nurse Education in Practice*, 71, 103716. https://doi.org/10.1016/j.nepr.2023.103716.

James, A.H., & Bennett, C.L. 2023. Power, politics and leadership. In Stanley, D., James, A.H., & Bennett, C.L. (eds), *Clinical leadership in nursing and healthcare*. 3rd edn. London: Wiley, pp. 385–402. 10.1002/9781119869375.ch18.

James, A.H., Carrier, J., & Watkins, D. 2021. Editorial: Nursing must respond for social justice in this 'perfect storm'. *Journal of Advanced Nursing*, 77(11), e36–e37. https://doi.org/10.1111/jan.14957.

James, A.H., Dimond, R., Jones, A., Watkins, D., & Kelly, D. 2024. Leading through the COVID 19 pandemic: Experiences of UK Executive Nurse Directors. *Journal of Advanced Nursing*, 1–13. https://doi.org/10.1111/jan.16329.

Mannion, R., Exworthy, M., Wiig, S., & Braithwaite, J. 2023. The power of autonomy and resilience in healthcare delivery. *British Medical Journal*, 382, e073331. https://doi.org/10.1136/bmj-2022-073331.

Marquis, B.L., & Houston, C.J. 2012. *Leadership roles and management functions in nursing*. 7th edn. Philadelphia, PA: Lippincott, Williams & Wilkins.

Ondaatje, M. 2012. *The cat's table*. New York: Vintage.

Popay, J., Whitehead, M., Posford, R., Egan, M., & Mead, R. 2020. Power, control, communities and health inequalities I: Theories, concepts and analytical framework. *Health Promotion International*, 36(5), 1253–1263. https://doi.org/10.1093/heapro/daaa133.

Ruger, J.P. 2020. Social justice as a foundation for democracy and health. *British Medical Journal*, 371, m4049. http://dx.doi.org/10.1136/bmj.m4049.

Valderama-Wallace, C.P., & Apesoa-Varano, E.C. 2019. Social justice is a dream: Tensions and contradictions in nursing education. *Public Health Nursing*, 36(5), 735–743. https://doi.org/10.1111/phn.12630.

Yoder-Wise, P.S. (ed.) 2015. *Leading and managing in nursing*. 6th edn. St. Louis, MO: Mosby.

CHAPTER 4

PERSONAL LEADERSHIP ACROSS THE CAREER
Developing your leadership mastery
Alison H. James

4.1 WHERE TO BEGIN ON THE LEADERSHIP LEARNING CONTINUUM

Throughout this book we argue that anyone can be a leader. As discussed in Chapter 1, traditional beliefs of leadership have been superseded by the realisation and understanding that people are not born leaders. Anyone can develop the skills needed to lead and influence. With this clear understanding, it is also important to know that, while some people want and plan to be leaders from early on in their careers, some arrive at leadership later, and that is also achievable. So whatever position you hold, whether you are a student or a chief executive, there is always much to *learn*, and everyone can lead effectively.

This chapter is subtitled 'developing your leadership mastery', but what do I mean by this? I would suggest *leadership mastery* includes the following:

- Having high levels of self-awareness
- Holding and wielding both cognitive and emotional intelligence with care
- Evidence of expertise and professional competence in the art and practice of leading
- Engagement skills within and across organisational systems
- A personal philosophy of career-long learning.

Learning is also an underlying theme in this chapter: to be skilled at something it must be fully understood; and to do this it is important to not stand still and to embrace a career-long learning approach to leadership. Alongside learning, we will also consider: the role of reflection and reflexivity; how emotions impact learning; how generational factors can influence; why empowerment is important and how mentorship and coaching can influence our leadership; and how to apply these support strategies to sustain ourselves and others as we influence those we work alongside.

In the earlier chapters I also discussed values and the importance of understanding your values and how they align with your profession and organisation. This is important as, to begin to fully develop as a leader, you should fully understand your values and how these drive you to find your leadership style or approach. Remember – values can change, so revisiting these through your career and personal life is an important self-awareness exercise (see Chapter 9 for Reflective Activities to help you with this). You will also find the chapter on emotional intelligence helpful as this is an important aspect of self-awareness and personal leadership, underpinned by your values base (see Chapter 5). As health and care professionals, our practice and ongoing learning are based on *reflection* and *reflexivity*. We will delve into both and find out how these strategies can support you and sustain your ongoing learning towards leadership.

DOI: 10.4324/9781003433354-5

> **Reflective Activity: 4.1**
>
> Think back to what you might consider significant learning experiences in your career, in your learning environments (such as university/college) or in clinical areas.
>
> What makes you consider this a learning point (or points)?
>
> Was it a challenging situation? Or was it to do with the people involved, someone you found inspiring or a role model or mentor, or perhaps a teacher or lecturer who inspired you and captured your interest?
>
> Try to recall what strategies you used to apply this learning to your practice. Was it reading and researching further about the issue; was it reflecting back and writing down what you learnt? You may have taken it a step further and researched the issue.
>
> What was it about this learning experience that made it so impactful? Write down all the aspects – whether it was the situation, the topic, the people or the learning strategies – and consider how you can continue to use these in your leadership learning.

4.2 IS EXPERIENCE THE NOBLEST WAY TO WISDOM?

In nursing and other healthcare journals there is much debate about the theory–practice gap that students experience when studying in the classroom and studying in practice, and how these align – or rather do not align – to support the student to learn effectively (James et al. 2022, Maben et al. 2007, Francis-Sharma 2016). After initial learning of course, we continue to seek additional learning opportunities in our professions to develop and gain further knowledge in our areas of interest and expertise, moving from novice to expert. This issue is therefore relevant across our careers and learning. When it comes to leadership development, this can also be challenging as what we learn about from reading and listening in a formal learning environment may not match what we experience in practice. This can be particularly evident when it comes to challenges for leaders. We may aim to be compassionate leaders; but, when faced with conflicts, challenging members of staff or power decisions made from the higher echelons of hierarchy, our aims may slide and we become pressured into behaviours or actions that do not align with our intended approach, or we may not be equipped with the strategies to cope with sudden challenges.

In my research of student nurses and how they perceive learning about leadership, an interesting finding was that some felt there were missed opportunities to critically evaluate experiences, explore the evidence and process their emotional response following an instance of seeing leadership in action (James et al. 2022). Effectively, the students felt they had little time to reflect, think on a deeper level and make sense of the experience. Of course, many theorists and educationalists have emphasised the importance of reflection in learning, and you will be familiar with many – such as Johns (2006), who states that reflection allows us to confront, understand and step towards resolving contradictions in our practice and in our values. So, it is disappointing if we are not providing our aspiring students with opportunities to do this in practice, and surprising if we are not continuing to apply this approach to our continuous learning.

Dewey's (1987) view of experience, reflection and cognitive processing of experience is the key to learning, rather than just experience alone. He considers reflection as enabling a consciousness that influences our experiences. If there is bias, prejudice or negative influences, this can obstruct positive actions that are underpinned by our vision or values. Reflexivity can enable the individual to critically transform. Polanyi (1964) supported this theory, believing that, with continued practice, discussion and analysis over time, students may come to understand the significance of an experience.

4.3   REFLECTION AND REFLEXIVITY

John Dewey was an American educationalist and philosopher who greatly influenced thinking in education in the twentieth century. Dewey's notions of learning were based on a pragmatic approach – namely that experience was a dynamic seam that accompanies all individuals, which is influenced by interactions and environments and is therefore constantly developing. An educative experience from which we learn something, according to Dewey (1987), is an experience where a connection develops between what we do and what happens as a consequence. Before we can learn with value, we must form the connection between the experience and the consequence, or outcome. Reflection is therefore a form of learning from experience, by doing and then reflecting on what happened. As the poet W.H. Auden states (2015, p. 44):

> we cannot be content merely to experience but must seek to make sense of it, to know what is its cause and significance, to find the truth behind … the basic stimulus to the intelligence is doubt, a feeling that the meaning of an experience is not self-evident.

The past and present are also important within this approach and influence actions in the future, notably focusing also on the location and how that influences the experience. Dewey describes continuity as an 'experiential continuum, meaning the construction of experiences on the quality of those situations (1987, p. 28). He was also interested in the aesthetic experience and its impact on learning, and I explore that further in Part 2 of this book, considering the arts and how we can use them to reflect and think on a deeper level about what leadership means.

Brockbank and McGill (2000) suggest that individual learning is influenced by our values and personal philosophies, and Chang and Daly (2012) link reflection to critical thinking and problem solving, so you can see how these reflective approaches link into areas of leadership we have discussed. Critical thinking and analysis are important in leadership because, to be an effective leader, it is essential to question assumptions, seek greater understanding of the issues, and enquire and seek knowledge and evidence before we act and make decisions. Becoming a reflective leader allows new knowledge and understanding to form and, if required, allows a change in behaviours (Jarvis 2013).

This is approaching 'reflexivity', a term which is often used in research to describe the process researchers take in self-critique and appraisal to evaluate their approach to the research process and how they can ensure awareness of their self-influence on the research. Reflexivity therefore goes one step further than reflection: it requires questioning of assumptions and norms and a wider consideration of social constructs, cultures, power and politics. I would define reflexivity as being active in seeking strategies and methods for questioning one's own attitudes and values as a leader, and seeking to further understand one's role in complex situations and influencing others. Critical theorists argue that reflection can be too self-absorbing; reflexivity leads to an awareness of 'false consciousness' prompting informed action or 'praxis (Habermas 1972, Carr & Kemis 1986, Rolfe et al. 2001). Being reflexive as a leader takes us a step forward in really understanding what effect we have on others, how we contribute to the social and professional structures of the cultures we work in, and how we are aware of our limits in knowledge.

Taking self-awareness and emotional intelligence to a deeper level through reflexivity, leaders can gain further insight into how their behaviours, their power, or the power and behaviours of others or of their organisational culture, influence others. Through reflexivity, leaders gain the ability to fully understand the space they practise in and their learning experiences, and how they analyse that learning to relate to others and shape accepted practice and ways of behaving. It almost becomes a superpower, recognising self-responsibility and how active it is in shaping the culture and surroundings, critically considering circumstances and relationships, considering their true values and vision and taking conscious action towards aligning these rather than reacting to experiences and circumstances without criticality (James 2023). Indeed, it is possible to experience the leadership of others where reflexivity is not evident, where leaders change their behaviours to suit other agendas, or where cultures within the workplace become toxic and practice becomes unsafe or unacceptable.

Analysis and introspection are also important in learning from errors. Making mistakes is of course common to us all; none of us will go through our professional lives without making a mistake, whether that is in decision making, action or non-action. How leaders manage and deal with mistakes is telling and highlights their integrity, trust, honesty and core values. How leaders respond to errors, whether their own or others', is important and gives others insight into their values. It can also demonstrate their approach to learning, either by approaching errors as a learning opportunity or as incidents to be managed and forgotten. Leaders who encourage an open culture of learning encourage staff to be accountable and responsible without fear of blame and retribution, which in turn supports trust (Jones & Kelly 2014, Bagot et al. 2023). By not dealing with issues of errors with consideration and scrutiny, the leader lacks the critical and analytical advantages of learning, both for those involved and for the organisation. It also offers further opportunity for repeating errors, so accountability, openness, fairness and quality standards are crucial in areas of patient care (Alingh et al. 2019). The benefits for leaders to view learning as an important value seem clear I would suggest, and it is certainly beneficial for our patients. If we can master reflexivity in our leadership, it is a significant skill to have.

There are many models of reflection that you will have encountered in your development as a professional, and all can support learning. Some of these are listed below, although you will find others that may be helpful:

- Johns (2006) – Johns' Model of Structured Reflection
- Rolfe et al. (2001) – Framework of Reflective Practice
- Mezirow (1981) – Model of Transformative Learning
- Gibbs (1988) – Gibbs' Reflective Cycle
- Schön (1987) – Reflection in and on Action
- Kolb (1984) – Kolb's Learning Cycle

Applying these models is an individual choice; you may prefer one over another or combine approaches. They are developed to support your ability to reflect and to be reflexive, so read around the topic and find a model that you can understand and that aligns with your approach to reflection and learning. For example, Mezirow's model can support critical reflection, and Gibbs and Schon provide a step and linear approach. A combination of approaches can provide advancement towards reflexivity facilitating deeper learning as you progress in your learning and development.

Reflective Activity: 4.2

Consider these benefits of reflection and reflexivity for leaders and write down examples of where you have experienced these in practice:

- **Empowerment** – Reflection can be empowering and emancipatory, supporting self-awareness.
- **Supporting team working** – Reflecting as a team can promote group learning and problem solving, and support a collective learning experience to improve patient care and outcomes.
- **Supports emotional intelligence and self-knowledge** – Developing self-insight requires a certain amount of reflection. Being aware of our actions, reactions and how we respond to others requires reflecting on experiences. Learning from those is important for leadership development.
- **Being clear about your values** – Stanley (2019) states that leaders who make their values clear to others and are positive role models for quality patient care are reflective in their approach.
- **Learning from mistakes** – Leaders who approach errors with openness, compassion, scrutiny and accountability encourage others to be trusting and accountable.

4.4   EMPOWERMENT

Empowerment is often defined as a process which enables individuals to develop a critical insight into their situation and their environment (Simmonds 1998), and a process which, through removing powerlessness, can enhance personal ability (Jones & Bennett 2018). Linked to context, feelings of disempowerment or powerlessness can be present in organisations where policies, structures and cultures inhibit individuals from expressing their beliefs and ideas (James & Bennett 2022). For example, the UK National Health Service (NHS) is a long-standing institution that clings to many traditional hierarchies and structures, with change often impeded by these traditional processes (Fisher & Kiernan 2019). Yet there is recognition of a need for change, which is evident in the growing initiatives for collective, distributive and compassionate leadership, and further driven by some of the most serious case reviews and reports into culture and leadership failings (Francis 2013, Andrews & Butler 2014). Senge (1990) defines a 'learning organisation' as one where people continually grow their capacities to create results they want to see; where innovation and new thinking are encouraged and nurtured, and new and expansive patterns of thinking are nurtured; where collective learning is encouraged and supported. So, while an organisation's need for and desire to change and adapt to new circumstances may be in the gift of some leaders, when dealing with vast organisations and complex systems this needs to be a collective drive and application of agency.

Western (2019) argues that empowerment can be manipulated to advance organisational needs or the individual needs of the leader; and the implication of empowerment can suggest the leader holds power over others, paternalistically giving permission for others to achieve self-empowerment. Other authors view empowerment as the process by which we can facilitate others to participate in decision making and encourage equality, reducing unequal power balances (Yoder-Wise 2015, Kreitner & Kinicki 1998). Paradoxically, Jones et al. (2000) also assert that empowerment can be bestowed by external agencies, as can sometimes be seen when we hear senior management claiming recognition for 'empowering staff' though processes such as development opportunities or reviews. Laschinger et al. (2010) links empowerment to improving patient care, which takes us back to values, and ensuring that, when empowerment is proposed, it is considered as part of improving patient outcomes or an individual's development, rather than as a gift. Considering how we learn and develop through empowerment, some perspectives view empowerment as an action that an individual has some control over in terms of their learning and development, rather than as a strategy used to impose empowerment on others.

Through teaching, encouraging, facilitating and directing, leaders can show a path to empowerment, but not actually empowering. Even if the policies and structures within an organisation are limited and the work and learning environment is the best it can be, it is still the individual's responsibility and choice to take that first step forward to empowerment. If they do not choose self-empowerment, they will not achieve it: "Empowerment isn't the path, it's the walk and the choice about which path to take" (James & Bennett 2022, p. 408). Enabling empowerment is central to the success of a leader and to effective accomplishment as a leader. This can become a legacy and culture of meaningful support for others if applied with thought and consideration of its impact. Influencing positive job satisfaction and staff retention is currently an imperative need to encourage individuals to choose and remain in healthcare professions. These have been found to be linked to feelings of autonomy, empowerment and agency (Gottlieb et al. 2021).

4.5   GENERATIONAL FACTORS AND LEADERSHIP

Our formative learning years shape our views of the world; and, as society changes and develops, generational groups are motivated by different values and expectations, and therefore respond to leaders differently (Reis & Blanchard 2022). Bennett et al. (2020) and James et al. (2024) explored nursing self-worth and perceptions of leadership, and state there has been a generational shift. Christensen et al. (2018) state that the nursing population is made up of Traditionalists (born between 1922 and 1945), Baby boomers (1946–1964), Generation X (1965–1979), Millennials (1980–1995) and Generation Z (born after 1995). Highlighting how the generational behaviours and expectations of nurse leadership vary, the authors state that the most significant number are Millennials, who are enquiring and seek opinions, valuing teamwork and problem solving, and expect feedback and value mentoring. Skilled in multitasking, they also expect a healthy work–life balance and a flexible approach.

Generation Z are described as realists, comfortable using digital technology in seeking knowledge and requiring less direction. However, they are often the most difficult to retain according to research in the UK and the US, and good pay and work conditions, flexibility and positive environments are expected (Holmes 2022, James et al. 2024). This applies across the professions as generational changes affect all aspects of society and culture. Generation Alpha (born 2010 onwards) will have been impacted by the COVID-19 pandemic, and are more likely to view diversity as a strength and positive aspect of society (Reis & Blanchard 2022). It is widely thought that, for leadership, an individual approach is more effective than grouping generations, as this makes assumptions and devalues the individual's capacity and drive for learning.

However, it is worth recognising for leaders and developing leaders that these generational groups do have trends and expectations, so being aware is always helpful and may support motivational techniques and strategies when it comes to teamwork. It is also helpful for organisations when thinking ahead about workforce planning. On an individual level, it can of course help individuals connect. However, as a leader, being aware and flexible when working with and supporting others is the best approach; and working with a mix of generations has huge rewards in terms of developing people skills and understanding what motivates staff.

4.6 THE ROLE OF EMOTIONS IN LEARNING TO BE A LEADER

Nayak (2016, p. 3) states: "Without emotion our perception is inferior." In my research on leadership development and student nurses, the experiences and emotional perceptions of role models, influencers, organisational cultures and hierarchical structures were clear themes. From emotionally positive influences, which were considered by students as inspiring and motivating, to negative influences, which had the opposite effect, all participants in the study had encountered and talked about examples of emotional events from experiencing leadership within clinical practice. The philosopher Martha Nussbaum (2008, p. 1) considers emotions as "geological upheavals of thought", which means emotions are not just impulsive reactions but intelligent perceptive responses to events and experiences, and form personal values and ethical codes.

Within healthcare, the actions and non-actions of practitioners have direct effects and impacts on others (James 2023). Therefore, as professionals who are accountable, we need to be fully emotionally conscious of choices and consequences (Rest & Narvaez 1994). Nussbaum (2008) also links emotional wellbeing to reasoning and decision making; and, in her discussion of political leaders and compassion, she has explored the application of compassion to conduct in public life, and the challenges of leadership and emotions in this context. While we may not wish our political leaders to be overly 'emotional' in its most basic sense, there are clear examples of successful political leadership where emotions are expressed and valued, for example by New Zealand prime minister Jacinda Ardern's resignation speech (McClure 2023). So, if we consider Nussbaum's view – that emotions are important in our rational judgements and value base – we can also infer that decisions made detached from emotions may push leaders further from their moral compass. There is also some evidence to demonstrate that emotions openly displayed by leaders influence their followers. For example, in business organisations, Nyland and Raelin (2015) suggest that followers may use the emotional messages conveyed by leaders to inform their decisions, which could have positive or negative consequences. Leaders may also manipulate their followers by appealing to their emotions.

Within the field of psychology, emotions are considered a series of psychophysiological changes in response to an event, and can include behavioural, expressive, physiological and cognitive responses. While research continues in the field of cognitive psychology, emotions are considered as influencing learning and performance in cognitive areas, learning and problem solving, self- motivation and regulation, and memory (McConnell & Eva 2015). The role of emotions in leadership therefore seems an important area for consideration, both in our response to them and our application of them in our decision making, and when they are conveyed by others.

Linking this aspect of learning back to reflection and reflexivity, this also seems to be an important consideration in that process – thinking about the emotions experienced either when you are the leader, making decisions and dealing with the consequences, or indeed when experiencing leadership from others, and the effect of that. How we apply this to our learning and development is an important part of developing personal leadership and mastery.

My research (James et al. 2022) also examined 'critical events' to explore the role of emotions. These critical events were experiences that altered perceptions and had an impact on the role of the research participants in practice, sometimes emotionally exposing the positive and negative, but prompting profound alteration in their views (Webster & Mortova 2007). Described as happening in areas or groups of practice where knowledge, culture and values may be shared, critical events can influence individuals' perceptions of themselves within their current role and what they aspire to be. Positive experiences of role models in leadership had constructive impacts, and students talked about positive leaders as being inspiring – with their approaches held in high regard and as best practice in leadership behaviour:

> Because there is a difference between having a mentor that wants to do it and a mentor that doesn't want to do it. And I've had both good and bad experiences … She said that a Band 6 [employee] is there not to progress themselves but to progress the people below them to, like, sort of, lift them up … if someone can lead you but without you realising that you're being led, is like, probably, the most effective way, I think, you don't even realise it … you just will always remember good mentors. (James et al. 2022, p. 6; slightly amended)

However, and interestingly, when negative leadership behaviours or experiences had an impact, this resulted in two responses. Some respondents stated they found it impactful as it made them realise how destructive it was on other staff and on them, so they made a concerted effort to be the opposite: "all the negative experience I've had has inspired me to be a good mentor and leader when I'm out there doing it" (James 2020, p. 94). Others felt it had a negative impact in making them feel inadequate and insecure:

> She was my mentor and a bully by all accounts. So that … for me it felt uncomfortable, intimidating. I wasn't supported. She was passive aggressive. And I could see it wasn't just me. But not a nice experience as a student. (James 2020, p. 118)

Here emotional response and how the individual reacts are important, for those who took a reflexive approach to learning, even when the event was negative, had made an important step in not taking the emotion as an inward response; rather, they determined to be inquisitive, explore the theory and use this to move forward in their leadership approach. They were applying the learning to inspire and be the opposite of that negative role model. Other research has found that role models are important for leadership development at all stages. For example, Stanley et al. (2022) assert that good clinical leaders are considered good role models; and role models can positively influence motivation to be effective and values-based leaders (Coventry & Russell 2021, Bender 2016).

Other theorists and writers in the area of leadership development have expanded similar approaches to apply as learning strategies that are helpful when we explore the effect of

---

Reflective Activity: 4.3

Try to recall a 'critical event' you have experienced. It might be how someone else was behaving and leading; and this could be an example of what you consider to be good leadership where values were clearly conveyed by that leader. It might be how they were communicating, or how they made decisions.

Think about your emotional response and what you could learn from the event.

Write this down and reflect on the incident (you could use a reflective model to support this).

Write down what you have learnt from that event, and what further reading could help you consider this on a deeper level of learning. What was it that was positive, and what else can you explore in terms of that approach? It may be that you can associate the behaviours with a leadership theory or style, such as congruent leadership, compassionate leadership or situational leadership (see Chapter 1). Write down why you make this association.

Now, what have you learnt about your own leadership approach from this exercise?

experiences. Craig et al. (2015, p. 47) call significant experiences 'crucibles', and encourage aspiring leaders to think about experiences that had a great impact and to focus on the learning from those. Bennis and Thomas (2002) also use the term to describe testing experiences that push individuals to their limit. This is another approach to acknowledging and scrutinising your emotions from an event that has great impact. For leaders this can become an effect method of reflection and reflexivity. This approach can also reframe your thinking and, with maturity and experience, can support your response and reaction. Rather than reacting, allowing time to process, consider carefully and really understand the situation. This approach also encourages you to think of such events without taking them personally and transforming a 'critical event' into a positive learning opportunity, which can strengthen your personal leadership and emotional intelligence.

4.7   COACHING AND MENTORSHIP FOR LEADERSHIP DEVELOPMENT

Coaching and mentorship can be highly effective in supporting leadership development and learning. As leadership is increasingly focused on nurturing human skills, relationships and development, innovation and improving care, coaching and mentorship centre on effective leadership development for individual as well as team performance. 'Action Learning' is also a highly effective, problem-solving and development technique, and we explore that further in Part 2 of this book.

Both coaching and mentorship are effective inherited skills, which means that, as you experience effective mentorship and coaching, you can also adopt these to support others in time and with experience. Coaching has been defined as: "Unlocking a person's potential to maximise their own performance. It is helping them to learn rather than teaching them" (Whitmore 2002, p. 8); and "Coaching is a human development process that involves structured, focused interaction and use of appropriate strategies, tools and techniques to promote desirable and sustainable change for the benefit of the coachee" (Cox et al. 2018, p. 1). Increasing individual agency and autonomy and providing psychological empowerment increases job satisfaction and morale, and coaching supports these in its motivational approach (Gottlieb et al. 2021, James & Arnold 2023). Coaching allows individuals to identify personal and professional goals in a safe and confidential environment, and to voice both personal and professional ambitions and self-identify a solution (Taylor & Webster-Henderson 2017). Key coaching skills include:
- listening to encourage thinking,
- asking powerful questions,
- paraphrasing and summarising feedback (van Nieuwerburgh 2020).

Coaching has been found to encourage self-focus, reflection and learning (Cable & Graham 2018). Access to coaching has been found to be highly effective in focusing on leadership development, and can be a significant support for your leadership development.

Mentorship can also be highly supportive, and finding a mentor who exhibits the style of leadership you aspire to be skilled in can provide insight into strategies and behaviours that may be helpful in your development. Mentors also foster positive cultures and, as mentioned previously, exhibit acceptable behaviours, values and ethics which can support not only individual development but also the culture within an organisation (Anderson et al. 2022). Table 4.1 outlines the differences between coaching and mentoring.

Table 4.1 Differences between coaching and mentorship

Coaching	Mentoring
Generally coaching lasts for a short duration, highly focused	Mentorship can be ongoing and can last for a long time
Consists of structured meetings, scheduled on a regular basis	Can be informal, meetings take place when mentee chooses
Focused on specific professional development goals and areas	A broader support and learning approach
Does not necessarily require the coach to have direct experience and knowledge or expertise of the coachee's area	Passes on experience and knowledge to the mentee and is usually more experienced and senior in the organisation
The agenda is set by the coachee, self-direction and goal setting	The agenda is set by the mentee; the mentor provides support and guidance for future roles
Includes specific personal development areas/issues, for example leadership skills and development	Can be inclusive of all areas for development and be less focused on one specific area

4.8 CONCLUSION

In this chapter we have considered topics and strategies that may be helpful to consider across your career, in your approach to learning and for your leadership development. The importance of career-long learning and the impact of emotions on learning, reflection and reflexivity have been discussed, as well as the role of empowerment and how generational differences may inform our motivation. As pioneering researcher and twice Nobel Prize winner Marie Curie, mentor and inspiration to many, said: "We must have perseverance and above all confidence in ourselves. We must believe that we are gifted for something and that this thing must be attained" (Curie 1937, p. 116). This chapter set out the importance of positive role models and presented suggestions for helpful support strategies, such as mentorship and coaching, to take forward for developing leadership mastery and confident leaders of the future.

REFERENCES

Alingh, C.W., van Wijngaarden, J.D.H., van de Voorde, K., Paauwe, J., & Huijsman, R. 2019. Speaking up about patient safety concerns: The influence of safety management approaches and climate on nurses' willingness to speak up. *BMJ Quality and Safety*, 28(1), 39–48.

Anderson, J., Dineen-Griffin, S., & Stanley, D. 2022. Creating a spirit of enquiry (enhancing research). In Stanley, D., Bennett, C.L., & James, A.H. (eds), *Clinical leadership in nursing and healthcare*. 3rd edn. Hoboken, NJ: Wiley, pp. 303–321.

Andrews, J., & Butler, M. 2014. *Trusted to care: An independent review of the Princess of Wales Hospital and Neath Port Talbot Hospital at ABMU Health Board*. Cardiff: Dementia Services Development Centre.

Auden, W.H. 2015. *The complete works of W.H. Auden*. Woodstock: Princeton University Press.

Bagot, K.L., McInnes, E., Mannion R., McMullan, R.D., Urwin, R., Churruca, K., Hibbert, P., & Westbrook, J.I. 2023. Middle manager responses to hospital co-workers' unprofessional behaviours within the context of a professional accountability culture change program: A qualitative analysis. *BMC Health Services Research*, 23(1), 1052. https://doi.org/10.1186/s12913-023-09968-6.

Bender, M. 2016. Conceptualizing clinical nurse leader practice: An interpretive synthesis. *Journal of Nursing Management*, 24, 23–31. https://doi.org.10.1111/jonm.12285.

Bennett, C.L., James, A.H., & Kelly, D. 2020. Beyond tropes: Towards a new image of nursing in the wake of COVID-19. *Journal of Clinical Nursing*, 29, 2753–2755. https://doi.org/10.1111/jocn.15346.
Bennis, W., & Thomas, R. 2002. *Geeks and geezers*. Boston: Harvard Business School Press.
Brockbank, A., & McGill, I. 2000. *Facilitating reflective learning in higher education*. Buckingham: Open University Press.
Cable, S., & Graham, E. 2018. 'Leading Better Care': An evaluation of and accelerated coaching intervention for clinical nursing leadership development. *Journal of Nursing Management*, 26, 605–612.
Carr, W., & Kemis, S. 1986. *Becoming critical: Knowing through action research*. Victoria: Deakin University Press.
Chang, E., & Daly, J. 2012. *Transitions in nursing: Preparing for professional practice*. 3rd edn. London: Churchill Livingstone.
Christensen, S.S., Wilson, B.L., & Edelman, L.S. 2018. Can I relate? A review and guide for nurse managers in leading generations. *Journal of Nursing Management*, 26(6), 689–695. https://doi.org/10.1111/jonm.12601.
Coventry, T.H., & Russell, K.P. 2021. The clinical nurse educator as a congruent leader: A mixed-method study. *Journal of Nursing Education and Practice*, 11(1), 8–18.
Cox, E., Bachkirova, T., & Clutterbuck, D. 2018, *The complete handbook of coaching*. 3rd edn. London: Sage
Craig, N., George, B., & Snook, S. 2015. *Discover your true north field book: A personal guide to becoming an authentic leader*. Hoboken, NJ: Wiley.
Curie, E. 1937. *Madame Curie: A biography, Part 2*. Da Capo Press.
Dewey, J. 1987. *The later works of John Dewey, 1925–1953. Volume 10: 1934, Art as experience*. Boydston, J.A. (ed.). Carbondale: Southern Illinois University Press.
Fisher, M., & Kiernan, M. 2019. Student nurses' lived experience of patient safety and raising concerns. *Nurse Education Today*, 77, 1–5.
Francis, R. 2013. *Report of the Mid Staffordshire NHS Foundation Trust Public Inquiry*. Norwich: The Stationery Office.
Francis-Sharma, J. 2016. Perceptions of leadership among final-year undergraduate nursing students. *Nursing Management*, 23(7), 35–39.
Gibbs, G. 1988. *Learning by doing: A guide to teaching and learning methods*. Oxford: Further Education Unit, Oxford Brookes University.
Gottlieb, L.N., Gottlieb, B., & Bitzas, V. 2021. Creating Empowering conditions for nurses with workplace autonomy and agency: How healthcare leaders could be guided by strengths-based nursing and healthcare leadership (SBNH-L). *Journal of Healthcare Leadership*, 13, 169–181. https://doi.org/10.2147/JHL.S221141.
Habermas, J. 1972. *Knowledge and human interests*. London: Heinemann.
Holmes, J. 2022. The NHS nursing workforce – have the floodgates opened? The King's Fund, 1 October. https://www.kingsfund.org.uk/insight-and-analysis/blogs/nhs-nursing-workforce.
James, A.H. 2020. *Perceptions and experiences of leadership: A narrative inquiry of leadership in undergraduate nurse education*. Doctoral thesis, Cardiff University. ORCA repository.
James, A.H. 2023. Valuing the emotions of leadership learning experience in nursing education. *Nurse Education in Practice*, 71, 103716 https://doi.org/10.1016/j.nepr.2023.103716.
James, A.H., & Arnold, H. 2023. Using coaching and action learning to support staff leadership development. *Nursing Management*, 29(3), https://doi.org/10.7748/nm.2022.e2040.
James, A.H., & Bennett, C.L. 2022. From empowerment to emancipation. In Stanley D., Bennett, C.L., & James, A.H. (eds), *Clinical leadership in nursing and healthcare*. 3rd edn. Hoboken, NJ: Wiley.
James, A.H., Kelly, D., & Bennett, C.L. 2024. Nursing tropes in turbulent times: Time to rethink nurse leadership? *Journal of Advanced Nursing*, 80, 8–10. https://doi.org/10.1111/jan.15766.
James, A.H., Watkins, D., & Carrier, J. 2022. Perceptions and experiences of leadership in undergraduate nurse education: A narrative inquiry. *Nurse Education Today*, 111, 105313. https://doi.org/10.1016/j.nedt.2022.105313.
Jarvis, M. 2013. *Beginning reflective practice*. 2nd edn. Andover: Cengage Learning.
Johns, C. 2006. *Engaging reflection in practice: A narrative approach*. Oxford: Blackwell.
Jones, A., & Kelly, D. 2014. Whistle-blowing and workplace culture in older peoples' care: Qualitative insights from the healthcare and social care workforce. *Sociology of Health Illness*, 36(7), 986–1002.
Jones, L., & Bennett, C.L. 2018. *Leadership: For nursing, health and social care students*. 2nd edn. Banbury: Lantern.
Jones, P.S., O'Toole, M.T., Hoa, N., Chau, T.T., & Pham, D.M. 2000. Empowerment of nursing as a socially significant profession in Vietnam. *Journal of International Scholarship*, 32(3), 317–321.
Kolb, D.A. 1984. *Experiential learning: Experience as the source of learning and development*. Upper Saddle River, NJ: Prentice-Hall.
Kreitner, R., & Kinicki, A. 1998. *Organisational behaviour*. New York: McGraw-Hill.
Laschinger, H.K.S., Gilbert, S., Smith, L.M., & Leslie, K. 2010. Towards a comprehensive theory of nurse/patient empowerment: Applying Kanter's empowerment theory to patient care. *Journal of Nursing Management*, 18, 4–18. doi:10.1111/j.1365–2834.2009.01046.x.

Maben, J., Latter, S., & Clarke, J.M. 2007. The sustainability of ideals, values and the nursing mandate: Evidence from a longitudinal qualitative study. *Nursing Inquiry*, 14(2), 90–113.

McClure, T. 2023. Jacinda Ardern says leaders can be 'sensitive and kind' in farewell speech. *The Guardian*, 5 April. https://www.theguardian.com/world/2023/apr/05/jacinda-ardern-leaders-can-be-sensitive-kind-farewell-speech-new-zealand.

McConnell, M., & Eva, K. 2015. Emotions and learning: Cognitive theoretical and methodological approaches to studying the influence of emotions on learning. In Cleland, J. & Durning, S.J. (eds), *Researching medical education*. Hoboken, NJ: Wiley, pp. 181–191.

Mezirow, J. 1981. A critical theory of adult learning and education. *Adult Education*, 32(1), 3–24.

Nussbaum, M.C. 2008. *Upheavals of thought: The intelligence of emotions*. 8th edn. Cambridge: Cambridge University Press.

Nayak, A. 2016. Wisdom and the tragic question: Moral learning and emotional perception in leadership and organisations. *Journal of Business Ethics*, 137(1), 1–13.

Nyland, P.A., & Raelin, J.D. 2015. When feelings obscure reason: The impact of leaders' explicit and emotional knowledge transfer on shareholder reactions. *Leadership Quarterly*, 26, 532–542.

Polanyi, M. 1964. *The educated imagination*. Bloomington: Indiana University Press.

Reis, J., & Blanchard, D. 2022. Gender, generational groups and leadership. In Stanley, D., Bennett, C.L., & James, A.H. (eds), *Clinical leadership in nursing and healthcare*. 3rd edn. Hoboken, NJ: Wiley, pp. 357–384.

Rest, J.R., & Narvaez, D. 1994. *Moral Development in the professions: Psychology and applied ethics*. Hillsdale, NJ: Lawrence Erlbaum.

Rolfe, G., Freshwater, D., & Jasper, M. 2001. *Critical Reflection for nursing and the helping professions: A user's guide*. Basingstoke: Palgrave Macmillan.

Schön, D.A. 1987. *Educating the reflective practitioner: Toward a new design for teaching and learning in the professions*. San Francisco: Jossey-Bass.

Senge, P.M. 1990. *The fifth discipline: The art and practice of the learning organization*. New York: Doubleday.

Simmonds, C.J. 1998. The rise of the supernurse is at the expense of others. *Nursing Times*, 94(37), 20.

Stanley, D. 2019. *Values based leadership in healthcare: Congruent leadership explored*. Los Angeles: Sage.

Stanley, D., Bennett, C.L., & James, A.H. (eds) 2022. *Clinical leadership in nursing and healthcare*. Hoboken, NJ: Wiley.

Taylor, R., & Webster-Henderson, B. 2017. *The essentials of nursing leadership*. London: Sage.

van Nieuwerburgh, C. 2020. *An introduction to coaching skills: A practical guide*. 3rd edn. London: Sage.

Webster, L. & Mortova, P. 2007. *Using narrative inquiry as a research method*. Abingdon: Routledge.

Western, S. 2019. *Leadership: A critical text*. 3rd edn. London: Sage.

Whitmore, J. 2002. *Coaching for performance*. London: Nicholas Brealey.

Yoder-Wise, P.S. 2015. *Leading and management in nursing*. 6th edn. St. Louis, MO: Mosby.

CHAPTER 5

BEING AN EMOTIONALLY AND SOCIALLY INTELLIGENT PROFESSIONAL

Mandy Brimble

5.1   INTRODUCTION

The aim of this chapter is to provide an overview of social and emotional intelligence and highlight their importance in providing compassionate leadership in the context of nursing and healthcare. Similarities and differences in social and emotional intelligence are discussed, as is the importance of appropriate empathy. Skills spanning the career trajectory and for specific stages are outlined and applied to leadership in a range of practice areas. Reflective activities are used to raise awareness of social and emotional intelligence traits in self and others, and the role of reflection in skills development is highlighted.

Social intelligence

The concept of 'social intelligence' was originally defined by Thorndike (1920). It is the ability to understand one's own feelings, thoughts and behaviours and those of other people (Goleman 2007). Success and failure in social settings aids the development of social intelligence. It is key to successful interpersonal interactions; hence it has also been identified as 'interpersonal intelligence' within Gardner's (1983) theory of multiple intelligences. People who are socially intelligent display core traits that help them communicate and connect with others, as shown in Table 5.1.

Emotional intelligence

'Emotional intelligence' refers to the ability to perceive, understand and manage one's own emotions and relationships. It involves being aware of emotions in oneself and others and using this awareness to guide thinking and behaviour. Emotionally intelligent individuals can

Table 5.1 Social intelligence traits

Effective Listening	Doesn't listen merely to respond but pays attention to what the other person is saying. Other people in the conversation feel they are understood and have made a connection.
Conversational Skills	Possession of conversational skills that enable the individual to carry on a discussion with practically anybody. They are tactful, appropriate, humorous and sincere. They remember details about people that allow the dialogue to be more meaningful.
Reputation Management	Mindful of the impression they make on other people. Considered to be one of the most complex elements of social intelligence. Managing a reputation requires careful balance. The individual must thoughtfully create an impression on another person while still being authentic.
Avoidance of Arguing	Understands that arguing or proving a point by making another person feel bad is not appropriate. The individual does not reject the other person's ideas but listens with an open mind, even when it is not an idea they personally agree with.

Source: Roshni (2023).

DOI: 10.4324/9781003433354-6

motivate themselves, read social cues and build strong relationships (Frothingham 2023). The emotional brain responds more quickly than the thinking brain. The amygdala in the emotional centre sees and hears everything that occurs to us instantaneously and is the trigger point for the fight or flight response. It is the most primitive survival response (Goleman 1995). Therefore, managing these swift, instinctive responses requires a high level of skill. Emotionally intelligent individuals demonstrate the following traits (Cherry 2023):

- An ability to identify and describe what people are feeling
- An awareness of personal strengths and limitations
- Self-confidence and self-acceptance
- The ability to let go of mistakes
- An ability to accept and embrace change
- A strong sense of curiosity, particularly about other people
- Feelings of empathy and concern for others
- Showing sensitivity to the feelings of other people
- Accepting responsibility for mistakes
- The ability to manage emotions in difficult situations.

Furthermore, the constructs of emotional intelligence outlined in Table 5.2 provide a clear overview of the concepts, how they can be defined and the type of competency into which each construct falls.

Although social intelligence and emotional intelligence are related, they are not the same thing. Emotional versus social intelligence can be thought of as the difference between how

Table 5.2 Goleman's constructs of emotional intelligence

Type of Competency	Construct	Definition and Characteristics
Personal (intrapersonal intelligence): knowing and managing emotions in oneself	Self-awareness	The ability to know one's emotions, strengths, weaknesses, drives, values and goals and recognise their impact on others while using gut feelings to guide decisions
	Self-regulation	Self-control, controlling or redirecting one's disruptive emotions and impulses; respond rather than react, think before acting; comfortable with ambiguity and ability to adapt to changing circumstances; trustworthiness and integrity
	Intrinsic motivation	A passion to work for reasons beyond money or status, awareness of personal motivators, optimism and perseverance in the face of adversity, organisational commitment.
Social (interpersonal intelligence): knowing and managing emotions in others	Empathy	Ability to understand other people's emotions and reactions (only possible if self-awareness is achieved), considering other people's feelings especially when making decisions
	Social skills	Managing relationships to get along with others, communication skills, finding common ground with others, building rapport, conflict management

Source: Adapted from Goleman (1998).

you relate to yourselves and how you relate to each other. When comparing emotional intelligence and social intelligence; emotional intelligence involves self-awareness, self-regulation and self-control. Social intelligence is less focused on one's own emotions or reactions, and more focused on sensitivity toward the feelings, moods and motivations of others and the ability to interact with others as part of a group (Positive Action 2023). Emotional intelligence has been identified as a key skill for effective and successful leadership (Goleman 1995), and both social and emotional intelligence are vital for managing interactions and relationships in healthcare roles (Lambert 2021) – especially those that involve emotional labour (Brimble 2021). More recently 'Knowing self', which comprises many elements of emotional intelligence, was identified as an enabler to healthful cultures in clinical practice (Dickson et al. 2023).

5.2   BENEFITS OF BEING SOCIALLY AND EMOTIONALLY INTELLIGENT

Possession of social and emotional intelligence can benefit an individual physically, emotionally, intellectually and socially in everyday life. For instance, increased self-awareness can lead to better physical health; social emotional skills can help reduce depression; intellectual curiosity can increase self-fulfilment through learning; and social skills can lead to positive interactions with others (Positive Action 2023). In healthcare practice these skills facilitate intuitive and respectful interactions with patients, which in turn builds trust and enhances patient care (Raghubir 2018). In addition, emotional intelligence can help healthcare professionals practise better self-care as they are more aware of what they are thinking and feeling (Dev 2019). Emotional intelligence therefore encompasses not only the ability of individuals to self-regulate responses to others but also to recognise when they need to take care of their personal emotional health. These aspects are key to leadership at whatever level the practitioner holds within their organisation's managerial hierarchy. The following section aligns social and emotional intelligence to leadership throughout the career trajectory.

Reflective Activity: 5.1 – Identifying social and emotional intelligence in self

- Write about a recent event at work involving three or more colleagues.
- What were your thoughts, actions and behaviours?
- What was your perspective on the issue?
- How was this influenced by your life experience, profession and values?
- Which social and emotional intelligence traits do you think you displayed?

5.3   USING SOCIAL AND EMOTIONAL INTELLIGENCE FOR LEADERSHIP THROUGHOUT THE CAREER TRAJECTORY

The student

Healthcare students often struggle to see how leadership applies to them. This is because they do not differentiate between leadership and management (Mutsa 2022) and interpret leadership to be a concept that only applies to those in hierarchical management positions. However, there are many ways in which a healthcare student can display leadership. For example, the UK's Royal College of Nursing (2024) proposes that a nursing student could demonstrate leadership by:

- Supporting, coaching or mentoring others, for instance through a buddy scheme for other students.
- Taking responsibility for own learning and development.
- Improving things for self and others by speaking out, for example as a cohort student representative at university.
- Advocating for a patient so their views can be heard.

All of the above are transferable to students of other healthcare professions and would require social and emotional intelligence traits to be effective.

The registered practitioner

In qualified healthcare practitioners these skills are also essential to everyday practice, as illustrated in the scenario and narrative in Box 5.1.

Box 5.1 Social and emotional intelligence in children's physiotherapy

A children's physiotherapist is asked to come to the ward to see a young child (who has cystic fibrosis) and their parent. The child has become very unwell because the parent has not undertaken the airway clearance techniques the physiotherapist has taught them on previous admissions.

The physiotherapist would inevitably be somewhat dismayed about the situation, and possibly a little exasperated. However, displaying these emotions would not benefit the child and the parent would likely feel judged, possibly reacting negatively and resisting further attempts to educate and support them. Therefore, with reference to Goleman's (1998) constructs of emotional intelligence, outlined in Table 5.2, the physiotherapist would need to be self-aware, recognise their own emotions and self-regulate, taking care that their behaviour did not reveal their feelings either through verbal or non-verbal communication. They would also need to remain motivated to working with the parent to improve outcomes for the child. Empathy for the child would be inevitable, but the practitioner would also need to ensure they use cognitive and compassionate empathy rather than emotional empathy as the latter can be counterproductive in helping relationships (Table 5.3). Social skills that span emotional and social intelligence would be key in this situation, not only for the practitioner to effectively communicate the airway clearance techniques and their importance but also, more importantly, to try to uncover the underlying reasons for the parent not complying with this part of the treatment regime.

By using emotional and social intelligence in these ways the physiotherapist is demonstrating leadership by advocating for the child, supporting the parent and showing them the best way to care for their child. They are being a role model for their own professional practice and for other members of the multidisciplinary team.

Table 5.3 Types of empathy

Type	Description	Desirability
Cognitive	Allows the individual to see a situation and the associated feelings from the other person's perspective. However, this type of intellectual understanding in isolation is primarily dispassionate.	Basic: useful in business meetings and negotiations
Compassionate	Enables the individual to feel 'for' the other person and elicits a desire to help or support. Essentially a middle ground between cognitive and emotional empathy, and described as the 'ideal'. The compassionate empathiser does not get 'sucked in' and take on the other person's feelings or burden; they simply understand, care and help.	Desirable: highly suitable for care situations
Emotional	Physically feeling alongside the other person, almost as if their emotions were contagious.	Highly undesirable in all situations, but particularly in care and helping relationships. Emotional empathy or empathy imbalance can lead to burnout and compassion fatigue. Professional behaviour can be compromised if self-regulation skills are poorly developed

Sources: Goleman (1995), Goleman et al. (2017), Cross (2019).

The team leader

Emotional and social intelligence have been shown to be key skills for effective leadership in terms of personal and professional success in healthcare (Prezerakos 2018, Stoichkova 2023). Although any person working in healthcare will interact with various individuals, those in senior positions will be required to understand and communicate with a significantly wider range of colleagues and members of the public, in many different situations (Skinner & Spurgeon 2005). The diversity of interactions involved in undertaking a senior healthcare position can be challenging; hence the importance of social and emotional intelligence in these roles. It is likely that this is why much of the literature applying these skills to healthcare focuses on those in team management positions. Nevertheless, this is useful in highlighting the demands of these roles and preparing those who seek career progression. For example, a study by Mansel and Einion (2019) of experienced senior nurses in the UK's National Health Service (NHS), holding Band 7 positions, found that emotional intelligence was a key factor in navigating the demands of their roles (Box 5.2).

Box 5.2   Emotional intelligence in nursing management

- Effective, strong leadership behaviours are needed to address quality of care issues in the NHS. Emotional intelligence (EI) is a key component in promoting effective, empathic leadership, which can enhance staff engagement, model

- empathic and emotionally intelligent behaviours and contribute to delivering more humanistic care.
- Leaders in this study were able to reflect some of the core values of EI within their management roles; but it was clear that a higher visibility of senior management was necessary to ensure a less hierarchical working environment.
- Significant difficulties were identified surrounding time, pressure and poor staffing levels, which meant that leaders were often unable to express EI behaviours. These factors would appear to suppress their potential in becoming effective EI leaders.

Challenges to acting in an emotionally intelligent manner while juggling the demands of a senior position were explored in the context of senior radiographers by Awwad et al. (2020), who found that increasing years of experience as a chief radiographer was associated with a reduction in some emotional intelligence constructs. This suggests that the pressures exerted by senior roles may erode emotional intelligence capabilities, as identified in Mansel and Einion's nursing study (final point in Box 5.2). Therefore, it is important that these skills are embedded from the start of a healthcare career so that they are the 'default' even when workplace pressures cause high levels of stress.

Reflective Activity: 5.2 – Identifying social and emotional intelligence in others

- Revisit the work event you reflected upon in Activity 5.1, but focus now on the words, actions and behaviours of your work colleagues.
- What did their perspective appear to be?
- Did it seem similar or different to yours?
- Why do you think it was similar/different?
- Which social and emotional intelligence traits could you identify in your colleagues?

5.4 USING REFLECTION AS A TOOL TO DEVELOP EMOTIONAL INTELLIGENCE

The reflective activities used in this chapter are informal and designed to be helpful for learning about social and emotional intelligence in yourself and others. It is no accident that reflection has been used here as a tool for self-exploration and exploration of others. As discussed, when identifying similarities and differences between social and emotional intelligence, some aspects are about what occurs within us and other aspects are about how we manage our relationships with others. While we can manage how we interact with others, we cannot control their thoughts and actions, only try to positively influence them via our behaviours. What we can influence is what we do to nurture our own interpersonal skills. Reflective thinking is a cognitive process whereby we examine our thoughts, feelings and actions to gain insight into and understanding of why we do what we do. Reflection can play a key role in developing emotional intelligence (Stanley 2022).

There are two fundamental types of reflection – 'on action' and 'in action' (Schön 1991). Reflection 'on action', i.e. after the event, enables us to identify positives and negatives that we can consider in making improvements in similar situations in the future. This enables us to become more self-aware, recognise triggers and think about strategies to manage emotions. It can also help us to appreciate the perspectives and emotions of others, i.e. by considering why they may have acted in a specific way. So, you can see that the reflective activities here were reflection 'on action'.

In contrast, reflection 'in action' occurs as events are unfolding. The ability to reflect 'in action' indicates that an individual has already developed a good level of emotional intelligence because pausing to think and make intentional choices about how to respond or proceed demonstrates self-regulation and self-awareness. Further strategies for developing social and emotional intelligence will be explored in Part 2 of this book.

5.5   CONCLUSION

This chapter outlines the key components of social and emotional intelligence, their similarities and differences. Different types of empathy are described, and the importance of using cognitive and compassionate empathy, but not emotional empathy, in professional caring relationships is highlighted. This is an important distinction in healthcare and is closely linked to the constructs of self-awareness and self-regulation in Goleman's (1998) model of emotional intelligence. Career-spanning and career stage-specific social and emotional skills have been highlighted using examples from practice and relevant research. Chapter 8 – entitled 'Becoming a self-aware professional: developing emotional and social intelligence' – revisits the concepts, theory and practice covered here. There this knowledge will be used to outline how social and emotional intelligence skills can be developed together with a career-spanning case study.

REFERENCES

Awwad, D.A., Lewis, S.J., Mackay, S., & Robinson, J. 2020. Examining the relationship between emotional intelligence, leadership attributes and workplace experience of Australian chief radiographers. *Journal of Medical Imaging and Radiation Sciences*, 51(2), 256–263.

Brimble, M.J. 2021. *How do children's nurses working in hospices manage emotional labour and professional integrity in long-term relationships with parents?* Doctoral thesis. Cardiff University.

Cherry, K. 2023. Emotional intelligence: How we perceive, evaluate, express, and control emotions. Available at: https://www.verywellmind.com/what-is-emotional-intelligence-2795423 [Accessed: 30 December 2023].

Cross, L.A. 2019. Compassion fatigue in palliative care nursing: A concept analysis. *Journal of Hospice and Palliative Nursing* 21(1), 21–28.

Dev, A. 2019. The importance of emotional intelligence in nursing. https://medely.com/blog/emotional-intelligence-in-nursing/#:~:text=Intuiting%20and%20respectfully%20interacting%20with,also%20for%20better%20self%2Dcare [Accessed: 20 January 2024].

Dickson, C.A.W., Merrell, J., Mcilfatrick, S., Gleeson, N., Westcott, L., Gleeson, N., & McCormack, B. 2023. Leadership practices that enable healthful cultures in clinical practice: A realist evaluation. *Journal of Clinical Nursing*. doi:10.1111/jocn.16951.

Frothingham, M.B. 2023. Emotional intelligence (EQ): Definition, components and examples. https://www.simplypsychology.org/emotional-intelligence.html [Accessed: 30 December 2023].

Gardner, H. 1983. *Frames of mind: The theories of multiple intelligence.* New York: Basic Books.

Goleman, D. 1995. *Emotional intelligence: Why it can matter more than IQ.* New York: Bantam.

Goleman, D. 1998. *Working with emotional intelligence.* New York: Bantam.

Goleman, D. 2007. *Social intelligence: The new science of human relationships.* London: Cornerstone.

Goleman, D., Boyatzis, R., Davidson, R.J., Druskat, V., & Kohlrieser, G. 2017. *Empathy: A Primer* (Building Blocks of Emotional Intelligence Book 6). Florence, MA: More Than Sound.

Lambert, S. 2021. Role of emotional intelligence in effective nurse leadership. *Nursing Standard*, 36(12), 45–49. doi:10.7748/ns.2021.e11782.

Mansel, B., & Einion, A. 2019. 'It's the relationship you develop with them': Emotional intelligence in nurse leadership. A qualitative study. *British Journal of Nursing*, 28(21), 1400–1408. doi:10.12968/bjon.2019.28.21.1400.

Mutsa, C. 2022. Students should be encouraged to pursue management and leadership. *Nursing Times*, 118(9), 12–13.

Positive Action. 2023. Social and emotional intelligence: An introductory guide. https://www.positiveaction.net/blog/social-and-emotional-intelligence [Accessed: 20 January 2024].

Prezerakos, P.E. 2018. Nurse managers' emotional intelligence and effective leadership: A review of the current evidence. *Open Nursing Journal*, 12, 86–92. doi:10.2174/1874434601812010086.

Raghubir, A.E. 2018. Emotional intelligence in professional nursing practice: A concept review using Rodgers's evolutionary analysis approach. *International Journal of Nursing Sciences*, 5(2), 126–130.

Roshni, M.J. 2023. Social intelligence. https://www.linkedin.com/pulse/social-intelligence-roshni-m-j/ [Accessed: 28 January 2024].

Royal College of Nursing. 2024. Leadership skills: How to demonstrate and develop leadership skills within your career. https://www.rcn.org.uk/Professional-Development/Your-career/Nurse/Leadership-skills#:~-:text=More%20examples%20of%20demonstrating%20your%20leadership%20skills&text=-Supported%2C%20coached%20or%20mentored%20others,services%2C%20resources%2C%20or%20costs [Accessed: 20 January 2024].

Schön, D.A. 1991. *The reflective practitioner.* Farnham, UK: Ashgate.

Skinner, C., & Spurgeon, P. 2005. Valuing empathy and emotional intelligence in healthcare leadership: A study of empathy, leadership and outcome effectiveness. *Health Services Management Research*, 18(1), 1–12.

Stanley, D. 2022. Reflection and emotional intelligence. In Stanley, D., Bennett, C.L., & James, A.H. (eds), *Clinical leadership in nursing and healthcare.* 3rd edn. Hoboken, NJ: Wiley, pp. 323–336.

Stoichkova, E.T. 2023. Emotional intelligence as the core of successful individual and professional performance of healthcare professionals. *Journal of Research in Humanities and Social Science*, 11(2), 172–177.

Thorndike, E. 1920. Intelligence and its uses. *Harper's Magazine*, 140, 227–235. https://gwern.net/doc/iq/1920-thorndike-2.pdf [Accessed: 30 December 2023].

CHAPTER 6

ADAPTING TO CHANGE

Clare L. Bennett

6.1 INTRODUCTION

Healthcare delivery is significantly influenced by political, economic and social landscapes that may impact the provision of resources and prioritisation of services. Drivers for change such as these are referred to as 'macro' changes since they operate on a level that is large in scale. For example, governments that oppose interventionist approaches may not prioritise public health services such as smoking cessation clinics or strategies that aim to decrease obesity. Yet with the election of new governments, health priorities and, therefore, policies and services are likely to change. Likewise, economic fluctuations and changes within communities, such as outbreaks of infectious diseases, can significantly influence resource allocation, which again will impact the delivery of clinical services.

Policy-level changes are not the only macro drivers for change in healthcare. Others may emerge from research findings that inform evidence-based practice. For example, in recent decades children were treated with aspirin; hospital patients were routinely turned every two hours, regardless of their particular risk of developing pressure sores; and a popular strategy for the management of diarrhoea was the 'BRAT' diet, which stands for bananas, rice, apple sauce and toast. However, following the emergence of research findings that questioned the efficacy and safety of such practices, evidence-based practice changed.

Additional drivers for change may be at the 'meso' or 'mid-range' level, such as the organisational level. Examples of meso drivers might be local procurement policies that lead to changes in the purchase of types or brands of equipment, such as pumps or monitors, that may require different modes of operation. Other meso drivers for change might relate to the demographics of the local population. For example, a healthcare organisation that serves an area with an ageing population could reduce services that are typically aligned with the needs of younger populations, such as sexual health services, and increase service provision to meet the requirements of older people.

Finally, drivers for change may also occur at the 'micro' or individual/small-group level. Such drivers are very familiar in nursing as they often reflect patient preference. For example, although oral medication for adults is usually administered in tablet form, if a patient struggles to swallow tablets it is standard practice for nurses to arrange for alternatives such as syrups to be provided. Similarly, care plans frequently change according to the unique progress a patient might make.

Change is therefore all around us in the context of healthcare. It may be planned, it may emerge gradually over time, or it may occur almost instantaneously. We therefore need to become expert at adapting to and leading change. However, this doesn't mean that we have to passively accept mandates for change; it is imperative that we first evaluate their value for patient outcomes.

DOI: 10.4324/9781003433354-7

Reflective Activity: 6.1

Think about what *change* means to you in relation to your personal life. How does it make you feel?

Now think about change in relation to your professional role. Write down how change can make you feel, and identify what factors make your perceptions of a particular change positive or negative.

Next consider how other healthcare professionals you have encountered appear to perceive and react to change. What factors influence their perceptions? Again, write these down.

6.2   RESPONSES TO CHANGE

Our responses to change are influenced by our individual life experiences and personalities as well as the characteristics of the change itself, how it is communicated and how the process of change is managed.

Positive adaptation to organisational change

During the COVID-19 pandemic, all aspects of healthcare provision were affected. Changes were rapidly implemented in a top-down approach with minimal negotiation. Many nurses were reallocated to unfamiliar care environments, and care provision changed due to the need for social distancing, the use of personal protective equipment (PPE) such as masks and visors, and the absence of family members to provide emotional support for loved ones. All of this was coupled with an increased demand for healthcare and the re-prioritisation of service provision.

Tort-Nasarre et al. explored hospital and community front-line nurses' responses to organisational changes during the COVID-19 pandemic in Spain through interviews with 23 nurses who provided care during the first wave (March to May 2020). The sample included 5 males and 18 females with a broad spread of ages. Quotes from participants included the following:

> Every day at 7 pm they told us what work we'd do the next day. We didn't know if we'd being doing respiratory care, wound care, house calls … Each day was different. We've been like this for 3 months. (Tort-Nasarre et al. 2021, p. 1987)

When they take me out of my department overnight and tell me, 'Starting tomorrow your department is closed; you're going to the COVID floor,' they don't tell me what will happen, what won't happen, how I should work, how I should protect myself. I start on my own to look at how it's transmitted, where I have to be more careful. Whether it's by medium-sized droplets, by contact … But [I did this] on my own. (Tort-Nasarre et al. 2021, pp. 1987–1988)

While recognising how stressful this time was for the nurses involved in this study, the authors reported that, despite the rapid nature of organisational change, the nurses successfully developed self-management strategies in the form of problem-solving, adaptation and learning. These strategies enabled the nurses to find solutions to the organisational changes they faced. Tort-Nasarre et al. also highlighted that personal resilience and social and institutional support can be supportive in protecting healthcare professionals against negative psychological outcomes during health disasters (Labrague et al. 2018, Cooper et al. 2020). However, effective leadership is also key (Labrague et al. 2021).

Resistance to change

In contrast to the example above, Cheraghi et al. (2023) assert that, while some nurses respond to change enthusiastically and view it as an opportunity to learn and grow, others will invariably be resistant to it. As you may have identified in Reflective Activity 6.1, some nurses might exhibit negative feelings towards change, such as frustration, alienation and sadness (Jones & Van de Ven 2016). In their integrative review, Cheraghi et al. (2023) identified that resistance to change is the result of a set of individual, interpersonal and organisational factors.

Reflective Activity: 6.2

Identify potential causes for resistance to change that focus on:

- Individual factors
- Interpersonal factors
- Organisational factors

Individual factors are difficult to predict as they are often unique to the individual. Cheraghi et al. (2023) identified that individual factors encompassed two sub-categories: (1) individual attitudes and perceptions; and (2) personality characteristics.

Individual attitudes and perceptions include:

- lack of awareness regarding the benefits of change
- negative attitudes, understandings and beliefs about change
- defensive feelings towards change that might give rise to fear, worry, frustration, anger, insecurity and confusion
- lack of trust
- fatigue
- feeling threatened
- lack of readiness to accept change.

Personality characteristics include:

- low motivation
- indifference
- inflexibility
- unfair judgement of change
- low self-confidence
- conservatism
- reluctance to move on from previous habits.

Cheraghi et al. (2023) further identified that *interpersonal factors* encompassed communication and cultural factors such as:

- colleagues' opinions
- communicating and expressing changes
- human relations (openness, mutual trust, loyalty)
- individual culture.

Finally, *organisational factors* encompassed three sub-categories: (1) management factors; (2) organisational values; and (3) structural factors.

Management factors include:

- a desire to strengthen the existing situation
- difficulty applying change
- organisational support
- lack of participatory management and not being involved in the change process
- limited appreciation and support
- speed of change
- lack of explicit feedback
- limited education and guidance.

Organisational values include:

- organisational culture
- negative organisational perception
- conflict with organisational identity.

Structural factors include:

- organisational characteristics
- resources and budget
- job properties
- environmental changes
- job characteristics.

An individual's resistance can be an obstacle to implementing change, so strategies that can address many of the factors outlined above therefore require careful consideration.

Reflective Activity: 6.3

Identify potential strategies that could reduce resistance to change that focus on:

- Individual factors
- Interpersonal factors
- Organisational factors

Nilsen et al. (2020) identified that change is more likely to be successful in healthcare organisations if healthcare professionals have the opportunity to influence the change, are prepared for the change and, importantly, value the change. Semi-structured interviews with 30 healthcare professionals employed in the Swedish system (11 physicians, 12 registered nurses and 7 assistant nurses) revealed the following:

- Changes that were initiated by the professionals themselves were considered the easiest and were rarely resisted.
- Changes that were clearly communicated and allowed time for preparation increased the chances for success.
- The need for and benefits of organisational changes needed to be communicated and understood.
- Organisational changes with clear benefits to patients were particularly valued.

Overcoming resistance

There are clearly many drivers of change as well as resistors, or factors that oppose change. One method of identifying the forces for and against change is through force field analysis, developed by Lewin (1947). Each force will differ in power, or force, which is represented in Figure 6.1 by the length and width of the arrows. For any change initiative to be successful, the forces that are driving change must be stronger than the forces resisting it.

As we have already seen in this chapter, the various forces will differ. The more obvious forces may centre on the availability of physical resources and finance, but the psychological and social responses of the people who are involved in the change can be of equal significance. By being aware of all of the resisting forces it is often possible to address and minimise them through discussion with the various people involved in the change.

Mutual trust between the change leader and those who are impacted by the change and/ or are involved in its implementation is more likely to elicit a positive response to new ways of thinking and working. Scholtes (1998) argues that trust is elicited through a combination of competency and caring, as illustrated in Figure 6.2. Competency on its own will bring about respect but not trust. Equally, if the individual feels cared for by the change leader but does not

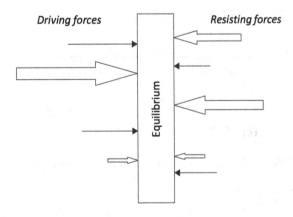

Figure 6.1 Driving and resisting forces

Adapted from Lewin (1947) (in Jones & Bennett (2018). Reproduced with permission from Lantern Publishing Limited).

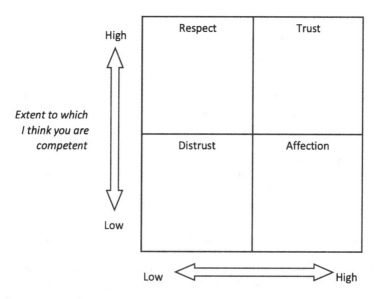

Figure 6.2 Competency, caring and trust

Adapted from Scholtes (1998) (in Jones & Bennett (2018). Reproduced with permission from Lantern Publishing Limited).

consider the leader to be competent or capable, it is likely that the individual will have affection for that person but may not trust them.

Reflective Activity: 6.4

Reflect on leadership scenarios where the leader has the trust of others. To what extent does Scholtes's (1998) model explain how they have achieved this?

6.3   WILL CHANGE LEAD TO IMPROVEMENT?

There is an implicit assumption that changes to service delivery will result in improvements. However, when we consider healthcare quality across the six domains of efficiency, safety, patient-centredness, effectiveness, timeliness and accessibility, some changes may in fact lead to compromised performance in one (or more) of these domains. It is therefore important that, prior to implementation, proposed changes are scrutinised for their potential impact on healthcare quality, including any unintended consequences (also known as unforeseen consequences or 'knock-on' effects).

In evaluating the potential impact of any change on healthcare quality, objective evidence is essential. Careful consideration of the potential unintended consequences of any change is also important. The Care Quality Commission (2023) effectively highlights how understaffing in the mental health sector, which is a change that has emerged over recent decades in the UK, can have a multitude of adverse, far-reaching impacts. For example, the safety of patients and staff can be compromised because a lack of therapeutic interventions can lead to an increased risk of violence and aggression. In addition, sustained staffing shortages are associated with the development of closed cultures, a lack of patient involvement in decisions about their care and patients' leave from in-patient units being cancelled.

Reflective Activity: 6.5

Imagine that you have been asked to lead the following changes:

- A reduction in the number of qualified nurses in a community nursing team
- A change in wound care procedures
- Updates to the clinical management of an infectious disease

How would you evaluate whether these changes are likely to positively or negatively impact the six domains of healthcare quality (efficiency, safety, patient-centredness, effectiveness, timeliness and accessibility)?

The reasons behind under staffing in healthcare are complex and politicians internationally often promise simplistic solutions. However, simple knee-jerk responses to any problem are often inadequate. Instead, a more thoughtful, far-reaching examination of the issue is required. The '5 Whys Technique' is a simple yet impactful problem-solving method that involves repeatedly asking 'Why?' to establish the root cause of a situation. The aim is to try to understand why a problem is occurring so that the correct solution can be identified, rather than simply making an assumption and potentially choosing the wrong intervention. An example could be that patients are consistently dehydrated on a ward. By asking 'Why?' repeatedly it might be identified that: drinks are not being made available to patients; cups are inappropriate; staff are not helping patients who require assistance; there is confusion among the team; misunderstandings might exist regarding 'Nil By Mouth' requirements; intravenous fluids might be routinely delayed, and so on.

Once all the potential reasons are identified, the team could then select the most likely reasons and interrogate these repeatedly. So, for example, if it is identified that the principal reason for patients being dehydrated is a delay in administering intravenous fluids, issues around the availability of suitably experienced and competent nurses to gain venous access and administer the fluids could be examined, along with factors around prescribing and the availability of the fluids themselves, along with pump availability and other relevant factors. After repeated examination, the root cause of the problem could then be identified so that appropriate strategies can be put in place to address the issue.

Reflective Activity: 6.6

Apply the '5 Whys Technique' to a problem that you have encountered in clinical practice. Examples might be discharge/referral delays, medication errors or poor nutritional intake, among others.

6.4   LEADING CHANGE

The US Institute for Healthcare Improvement (2024) highlights that, "While all changes do not lead to improvement, all improvement requires change. The ability to develop, test, and implement changes is essential for an individual, group, or organization that wants to improve."

Change management and quality improvement models provide guiding principles for change. This part of the chapter introduces several key models that you may find helpful in guiding you in leading change in practice. Although the models are presented separately, several complementary models can be used together.

Kotter's eight-stage change process

John Kotter's (1996) process is as follows:

1) Establish a sense of urgency.
2) Involve people at all levels to construct a shared vision and address specific needs.
3) Develop a vision and strategy that work towards the planned change.
4) Communicate the change/vision to others.
5) Empower employees for action.
6) Strive for short-term wins.
7) Consolidate gains and produce more change.
8) Anchor new approaches in the culture.

It is important to note that stage 8 of this model is frequently overlooked and requires just as much energy as the earlier stages.

Beckhard and Harris's change equation

Beckhard and Harris's (1987) model prioritises staff engagement, with an equation offering a solution to resistance encompassing dissatisfaction (D) with the present situation, a vision (V) for what can be achieved and the first steps (F) taken towards the vision. Cumulatively these can overcome resistance (R). The model is expressed as:

$$D \times V \times F > R$$

In keeping with fundamental mathematical principles, if any one of the three components is overlooked, and therefore yields zero, the resistance to change will not be overcome. This model is particularly useful when planning the change to ensure that the three elements are addressed, as well as during the change process as a problem-solving tool to establish why resistance to the change may be occurring.

The Model for Improvement

The most widely known approach to quality improvement is the Model for Improvement, which commences with the following three key questions:

1) What are we trying to accomplish?
2) How will we know that the change will be an improvement?
3) What change can we make that will result in an improvement?

Once these questions have been considered and answered, the next stage is implementation of the Plan–Do–Study–Act (PDSA) cycle:

• **Plan:** Agree on objectives, predict outcomes, plan the who/what/when/where/how and plan data collection.

- **Do:** Carry out the change, document all observations, collect and record data.
- **Study:** Conduct data analysis, compare results with predictions, compile a summary of insights and knowledge gained.
- **Act:** Identify what changes need to be made for the next PDSA cycle.

Reflective Activity: 6.7

Think through how you would use the Model for Improvement to achieve increased compliance with handwashing standards among all staff on a hospital ward. First outline:

1) What you are trying to accomplish
2) How you will know that the change is an improvement
3) What change you will make that will result in an improvement.

Then:

- **Plan:** Agree on objectives, predict outcomes, plan the who/what/when/where/how and plan data collection.
- **Do:** Carry out the change, document all observations, collect and record data.
- **Study:** Conduct data analysis, compare results with predictions, compile a summary of insights and knowledge gained.
- **Act:** Identify what changes need to be made for the next PDSA cycle.

Lewin's three-stage process of change

Lewin (1951) advocates a planned approach to change using three stages – 'unfreezing', 'movement' and 'refreezing':

- 'Unfreezing' is concerned with enabling the team to recognise the need for change, and challenging and reducing the forces that support established ways of working.
- 'Movement' is the phase where new attitudes and/or behaviours are developed and the organisation moves through the various stages of implementation of the change.
- 'Refreezing' is characterised by ensuring that the change is sustained. The change is reinforced through supportive mechanisms, such as coaching, appropriate policies and organisational norms.

Cummings and Worley's six guidelines for cultural change

With parallels to Kotter's eight-step change model, Cummings and Worley (2005) propose the following guidelines specifically for cultural change:

1) Devise and articulate a clear strategic vision.
2) Display a willingness to change on the part of senior management.
3) Model the cultural change at the highest level within the organisation.
4) Alter the organisation to support organisational change.
5) Select and socialise newcomers and bypass those who do not fit in.

6) Develop an understanding of the ethical and legal issues that may arise as a result of the cultural change.

Cultural change is widely considered to be the most challenging of changes and requires organisational commitment for its achievement.

6.5   IT TAKES MORE THAN A MODEL

While the above models provide guidance, they will be of little benefit to you as a change leader unless you are able to fully utilise your leaderships skills in motivating colleagues, negotiating and communicating effectively. Clear, consistent, regular two-way communication is essential in facilitating change. Likewise, the ability to motivate others is another key.

Motivational theory

McClelland (1987) identifies three types of motivational need:

- achievement motivation
- authority/power motivation
- affiliation motivation.

Each of these can be appealed to throughout the change cycle, with different aspects of the process being highlighted to different individuals, depending upon their motivational needs. For example, a colleague who values affiliation may be motivated to engage in a particular change project to cultivate relationships, in which case this aspect of the project can be emphasised during the planning stage of the change process. Similarly, those who are motivated by achievement may find that particular aspect of a change project motivational.

Herzberg's (1966) motivational theory asserts that certain factors ('motivators') truly motivate people, whereas others ('hygiene factors') only temporarily drive them. 'Motivators' include a sense of achievement, recognition, the work itself, responsibility, advancement and personal growth. 'Hygiene factors' or 'maintenance factors' centre on status, security, company policy and administration, supervision, personal life, salary, work conditions and relationships with subordinates, peers and supervisors. People might be unhappy if their hygiene needs are not met; but once they are satisfied, the sense of satisfaction is only temporary. Herzberg therefore suggests that people will not be 'motivated' by the satisfaction of 'hygiene' needs. However, all of the 'motivators' can be readily addressed throughout the change process as long as the leadership style is sufficiently sensitive to allow for this.

Negotiating skills

Most changes require some degree of negotiation. Successful negotiation leads to an outcome that both parties are fully committed to and feel they benefit from. 'Principled negotiation' (Fisher & Ury 1981) is widely regarded as an ethical and productive approach to negotiation.

The process begins with those engaged in the negotiation defining the issue or problem together. The first principle is *Separate the people from the problem*. The aim is to be resolute with the problem but respectful to the individuals involved in the discussions. For example, if the problem is that an adequate supply of equipment is not consistently available in a department, the normal line the discussion may take is to blame the staff who have placed the order. The discussions may even become personal. However, in separating the people from the problem, the focus will be on the processes rather than the individual(s). That is not to say that staff are not accountable for their actions; but they are treated with respect and the issue is explored from all angles.

The second principle is *Focus on interests, not positions*. Taking up a particular position – for example 'I will only accept …' or 'I will not …' – will often lead to an impasse. However, even when opposing positions are adopted there are often still shared and compatible interests that can be explored, such as the desire to deliver a high-quality service. To identify shared interests, questions such as 'Why?' and 'Why not?' can be effective.

The third principle, *Invent options for mutual gain*, is something that can be explored prior to meeting; however, this process can also be beneficial if carried out within the negotiations. In looking for 'mutual gain' it can be beneficial to identify shared interests.

The fourth principle, *Insist on objective criteria*, requires preparation in that the 'objective criteria' may concern issues such as professional standards, accepted practice, the evidence base, efficiency, costs, or law and ethical standards that may need to be explored in some detail.

Reflective Activity: 6.8

Imagine you want to negotiate funding for a training programme for a group of nurse colleagues. Consider how you would apply the four areas of principled negotiation outlined above:

1) Separate the people from the problem.
2) Focus on interests, not positions.
3) Invent options for mutual gain.
4) Insist on objective criteria.

6.6   SUMMARY

Change can be exciting, daunting, uplifting, depressing … in other words it can elicit highly emotional responses within individuals and teams. By listening to colleagues' perspectives, evaluating whether the proposed change is the 'right' change and working systematically and supportively, the change process is more likely to have a positive outcome for all involved and, in particular, patients and their loved ones.

REFERENCES

Beckhard, R., & Harris, R. 1987. *Organizational transitions: Managing complex change*. 2nd edn. Boston: Addison-Wesley.

Care Quality Commission. 2023. Monitoring the Mental Health Act in 2021 to 2022. https://www.cqc.org.uk/publications/monitoring-mental-health-act/2021-2022/staff-shortages [Accessed: 1 February 2024].

Cheraghi, R., Ebrahimi, H., Kheibar, N., et al. 2023. Reasons for resistance to change in nursing: An integrative review. *BMC Nursing*, 22, Art. 310. https://doi.org/10.1186/s12912-023-01460-0.

Cooper, A.L., Brown, J.A., Rees, C.S., & Leslie, G.D. 2020. Nurse resilience: A concept analysis. *International Journal of Mental Health Nursing*, 29(4), 553–575. https://doi.org/10.1111/inm.12721.

Cummings, T.G., & Worley, C.G. 2005. *Organization development and change*. Cincinnati OH: South-Western College/Thomson Learning.

Fisher, R., & Ury, W. 1981. *Getting to yes: Negotiating agreement without giving in*. London: Hutchinson Business.

Herzberg, F. 1966. *Work and the nature of man*. London: Crosby Lockwood Staples.

Institute for Healthcare Improvement. 2024. Model for improvement: Selecting changes. https://www.ihi. org/resources/how-to-improve/model-for-improvement-selecting-changes#:~:text=While%20all%20 changes%20do%20not,organization%20that%20wants%20to%20improve [Accessed: 1 February 2024].

Jones, S.L., & Van de Ven, A.H. 2016. The changing nature of change resistance: An examination of the moderating impact of time. *Journal of Applied Behavioral Science*, 52(4), 482–506.

Jones, L., & Bennett, C. 2018. *Leadership for nursing, health and social care students*. 2nd edn. Banbury: Lantern.

Kotter, J. 1996. *Leading change*. Cambridge, MA: Harvard Business School Press.

Labrague, L.J., Lorica, J., Nwafor, C.E., & Cummings, G.G. 2021. Predictors of toxic leadership behaviour among nurse managers: A cross-sectional study. *Journal of Nursing Management*, 29, 165–176. https://doi. org/10.1111/jonm.13130.

Labrague, L.J., McEnroe-Petitte, D.M., Leocadio, M.C., Van Bogaert, P., & Cummings, G.G. 2018. Stress and ways of coping among nurse managers: An integrative review. *Journal of Clinical Nursing*, 27(7–8), 1346–1359. https://doi.org/10.1111/jocn.14165.

Lewin, K. 1947. Frontiers in group dynamics: Concept, methods and reality in social science; social equilibrium and social change. *Human Relations*, 1(1), 5–41.

Lewin, K. 1951. *Field theory in social science: selected theoretical papers*. Cartwright, D. (ed.). New York: Harper & Row.

McClelland, D.C. 1987. *Human motivation*. Cambridge: Cambridge University Press.

Nilsen, P., Seing, I., Ericsson, C., et al. 2020. Characteristics of successful changes in health care organizations: An interview study with physicians, registered nurses and assistant nurses. *BMC Health Services Research*, 20, Art. 147. https://doi.org/10.1186/s12913-020-4999-8.

Scholtes, P. 1998. *The leader's handbook: Making things happen, getting things done*. New York: McGraw-Hill.

Tort-Nasarre, G., Alvarez, B., Galbany-Estragués, P., et al. 2021. Front-line nurses' responses to organisational changes during the COVID-19 in Spain: A qualitative rapid appraisal. *Journal of Nursing Management*, 29, 1983–1991. https://doi.org/10.1111/jonm.13362.

CHAPTER 7

LEADERSHIP AND WELLBEING
An achievable challenge or impossible dream?

Teena J. Clouston

7.1   INTRODUCTION

The relationship between being a leader in health and social care and personal wellbeing is an interesting one. My research in this field has suggested it is a rather invidious affair, with the responsibilities of the position frequently conflicting with achieving a sense of wellbeing for various reasons. Factors such as compromising personal time and energy to meet work expectations, ethical and moral dilemmas resulting in cognitive dissonance and challenges to personal integrity are all regular contenders (Clouston 2014, 2015). These can result in increased stress and ultimately burnout, both associated with a loss of meaning and purpose in life. Of course everyone's experience is different, perspectives vary and what we want from life is individually modulated. However, if you are a leader and working in health and social care, you are likely to find some something here that reflects your lived experience. We will start by discussing the concept of wellbeing; then consider the challenges for leaders in attaining this, followed by some strategies that can actually be implemented to help sustain wellbeing in the workplace.

7.2   WHAT IS WELLBEING?

To begin, let's consider what we understand by the concept of 'wellbeing'. Interestingly, the term itself is not as easy to comprehend as you might think; this is because it comprises multiple layers. First, it is associated with human flourishing experienced though purposefulness and a sense of meaning in life at both subjective and societal levels (Clouston 2015, Coultard et al. 2018). Second, it is frequently correlated with good health, quality of life, resilience and sustainability at the micro, meso and macro levels (World Health Organization (2023). Wellbeing thus functions as a system and, consequently, personal or subjective wellbeing cannot exist in a vacuum *because* it is influenced by the socio-cultural and economic context in which the individual is situated.

Subsequently, in the milieu of leadership and wellbeing, we have to consider how society influences the culture of the workplace and then how that, in turn, impacts on the individuals who work in it. For example, economic and environmental determinants in the system can influence an individual's ability to experience autonomy and satisfaction and achieve a sense of meaning and purpose in work and/or life (Clouston 2015). Because these interconnected forces form the landscape and lived experience of wellbeing, the focus of this chapter is structured around the subjective nature of wellbeing in dialogue with the organisational and wider social context. Only by viewing it in this way can we consider the personal and practical skills you can utilise and develop to support you to survive within that milieu. Let's begin by reviewing what we mean by subjective wellbeing.

7.3   SUBJECTIVE WELLBEING

Within the literature there is some general agreement that wellbeing, as a personal experience, is something that is both subjective and meaningful to the individual. The philosophical terms 'hedonistic' and 'eudemonic' are frequently used to describe a sense of positive feeling and

DOI: 10.4324/9781003433354-8

meeting one's full potential in life, respectively (Webb 2023). Encompassing these two elements, Simons and Baldwin (2021, p. 990) suggest the following definition for personal wellbeing: "Wellbeing is a state of positive feelings and meeting full potential in the world. It can be measured subjectively and objectively using a salutogenic approach." 'Salutogenesis' is a term used by Antonovsky (1987, 1996) to describe the presence of a personal *sense of coherence*, which he argued underpins the ability to achieve and maintain wellbeing. This is a dispositional trait or ability that is marked by three key qualities: (1) meaningfulness, (2) comprehensibility and (3) manageability.

The presence of meaningfulness

Antonovsky (1996) defined this as a psychological quality and way of being that is marked by the ability to maintain a positive outlook, motivation and drive to progress while moving forward, even in stressful or challenging situations. People who have these attributes are solution focused and see life challenges as opportunities to develop, as opposed to barriers to prevent growth or progress (Galletta et al. 2019). These are, if you like, people whose glass is half full, not half empty.

A sense of comprehensibility

Antonovsky (1996) maintained that individuals with this quality have the cognitive abilities to understand and make sense of the challenges or situations around them. The idea here is that when people can make sense of what is happening, they can address it more pragmatically and apply solutions or strategies to improve or resolve it. Now that, of course, is a valuable skill for leaders, who, theoretically, require the ability to solve problems, make informed decisions and address situations as they arise.

The quality of manageability

Finally, manageability is an instrumental or practical skill; it is about having sufficient external and internal resources to cope with adverse events or challenges (Eriksson & Mittelmark 2017). This is an interesting one because, to achieve this, leaders require not only a personal but also a professional and/or organisational sense of control and autonomy, as well as access to available resources to address challenges as required. This means that a personal sense of coherence is not only about a sense of positivity and meaningfulness, cognisance and decision-making abilities; it is also about having access to and autonomy over resources to address everyday problems. This is really important in an organisational workplace context because ownership and power over resources frequently lie with the organisation, not the individual. Thus personal agency over those determinants can be limited in terms of pragmatic or meaningful change (Simons & Baldwin 2021). For leaders, who are challenged to drive culture change, improve performance and staff wellbeing, this can be a real issue.

Reflective Activity: 7.1

Think about your understanding of the three qualities that create a sense of personal coherence.

Write these down.

Reflect on your personal sense of wellbeing and what is meaningful to you in everyday life.

7.4   THE CHALLENGES OF ACHIEVING AND MAINTAINING WELLBEING AS LEADERS

The trouble with being a leader is that your role often requires you to address and maintain the health and wellbeing of your staff and meet organisational outcomes such as efficiency, effectiveness and performance targets. As the levels of stress and burnout rise in health and social care staff, and as organisational cultures and leadership styles are implicated, so the pressures on leaders increase to address these. If this externally modulated pressure were not enough, there is also your own health and wellbeing to consider, which tends to lie unheeded while you do the job and strive to balance meeting both organisational diktats and staff wellbeing.

Values-based models of leadership are presently being heralded as a means to achieve not only organisational outcomes but also to sustain the wellbeing of all staff, including leaders. Although more implementation and research are needed to support this assertion, some evidence suggests that these approaches, if successfully executed, can be effectual in improving both organisational effectiveness and staff wellbeing (e.g., Bailey & West 2022, West 2021). However, these styles of leadership are not naturally occurring in health and social care. Research has shown that existing cultures are performance-driven, utilising models of power and control, fear and insecurity, and focusing on performance over wellbeing – all promoted by neoliberal ideals (Clouston 2014, 2015).

Neoliberalism is a perverse and powerful driving force in global constructs of work. It promotes paid work as the essential activity for all adults, and ensures that the organisation controls the workforce in order get the best out of employees (Clouston 2015). Its focus on performance creates a 'more with less' culture though which staff are expected to achieve greater outcomes with less money, staff and equipment. It causes division by supporting a focus on individualism and eroding collective decision making. Further, it denigrates staff wellbeing to focus on productivity and financial growth. This kind of thinking and rationalisation does not support wellbeing; instead it fosters work–life imbalance and increases stress, burnout, compassion fatigue and rust-out – i.e., disengaged staff who are apathetic and cynical in the face of adverse organisational conditions (Clouston 2015).

In this kind of environment, and without a root and branch approach to change, leaders can find themselves fighting against intransigence and toxic cultures that can lead to a sense of increased stress and pressure (Clouston 2015). This can create ethical dilemmas for leaders who try to deal with conflicting principles and values while also trying to maintain elements of their own personal and professional integrity in how their values are lived and enacted ontologically.

Values-based leadership models attest that, by addressing the ethical, moral and practical nature of leaders, as well as the strategic skills and practice of leadership, leaders can overcome some of these dilemmas and create workplace cultures that value staff. Strategies to achieve this include: empowering staff and long-term value creation (Caldwell & Anderson 2020); fostering high levels of trust, authenticity and integrity marked by congruence between values, beliefs and actions (Stanley 2022); and providing employees with the resources to nurture and achieve success (Denier et al. 2019). The problem at the time of writing is that while these models are emerging, they remain liminal in many settings. Thus, even leaders who have nurtured the qualities to achieve and sustain personal wellbeing, such as a personal sense of coherence, can find themselves sinking. So, what can you do to influence the lived experience of wellbeing while organisational cultures catch up?

Reflective Activity: 7.2

Think of the qualities and approach you currently use in your workplace.
Write these down.
Reflect on how these 'fit' with the organisational attributed and practised values and approaches.

7.5 STRATEGIES TO IMPROVE WELLBEING FOR SELF AND OTHERS

The following steps are practical strategies for addressing and maintaining personal wellbeing both in work and everyday life. While they focus on personal wellbeing, they do consider the influence of the situated organisational context. Please note that these strategies are interconnected and dynamic; they do not have to be followed in the order given. Start with the one that speaks to you the most, or the one that feels achievable in your unique context and situation. Think about how these strategies fit with Antonovsky's (1996) notion of personal coherence as you work through them. This will enable you to review your own personal attributes and dispositions in terms of wellbeing as well as offer some practical solutions to improve them. Table 7.1 provides a brief summary to remind you of them.

Step 1: Living life in balance

Having sufficient resources to meet personal life commitments successfully, or are least satisfactorily, is critical skill to achieving a sense of personal wellbeing. As we have discussed, the neoliberal workplace can be greedy, and will take more time and energy from you if it can. Although all models of values-based leadership aim to address this, the lived experience in most health and social care workplaces remains predicated on a performance-driven model that takes time and energy from staff rather than addressing their wellbeing (Clouston 2015). So, what can you do to try and support both yourself and your staff in terms of a balanced lifestyle as we transition to a more values-based culture?

Table 7.1 Antonovsky's (1996) sense of personal coherence

The presence of meaning in life	Living with integrity, having a positive outlook, high levels of motivation and drive to progress and move forward, even in times of stress or challenge. People with this quality are solution-focused and see life challenges as opportunities rather than barriers (Galletta et al. 2019).
Sense comprehensibility	Having the cognitive ability to understand and make sense of the challenges or situations around you. The notion here is that when people can make sense of what is happening, they can address matters pragmatically and apply solutions or strategies.
The quality of manageability	An instrumental or practical skill marked by having sufficient external and internal resources to cope with adverse events or challenges (Eriksson & Mittelmark 2017). In essence this requires a sense of control and autonomy as well as access to available resources to address challenges.

Balance your personal resources of time and energy

The analogy of the 'Ship of Life' is a really useful way of reviewing how you are actually using your personal resources of time and energy in your everyday life. If you look at the example in Figure 7.1 you will see that this individual works and has caring and home responsibilities, but also has time for rest, leisure and social activities as well as spending time in nature and just 'being' – both of which, for them, are personally meaningful activities.

This is a healthy life balance, with a diverse mix of activities that are both taking and giving energy, thus supporting wellbeing because there are both restorative and depleting activities. Moreover, because there is a spectrum of activities in this person's life, when there is a problem in one area (say, work) the other activities will hopefully help keep the person afloat.

Look again at the Ship of Life in Figure 7.1. Imagine that work expanded to take up most of the cargo hold, with only leisure left. What do you think would happen if work became badly disrupted or a problem occurred? Well, when one activity dominates and that situation becomes unstable, the impact on personal wellbeing can be devastating because the individual will feel totally overwhelmed and 'sink'.

So, let's have a look at your life balance. Let's start by drawing your own Ship of Life. You can then share the idea with your staff to help them reflect on their life balance. The process is a simple one. Imagine yourself as a ship, and place all the different activities you do every day in the hold. Look at the example in Figure 7.1 to help you do this. Each individual cargo hold will look different depending on the person because it reflects their personal interests and commitments. Once you have completed your ship, think about whether anything is missing from your cargo hold. Is there anything you would like to be doing that you have lost or compromised to achieve the things you feel you have to do every day? The strategy of compromising or 'letting go' of certain activities – usually the ones you enjoy most, such as interests or social activities – is a common way of coping with busyness and prioritising the things you feel you *have* to do, like work and personal commitments, over the things you *want* to do (Clouston 2015).

Now, while this strategy may appear to help in managing expectations and commitments, it does very little for wellbeing. A well-balanced life must include a variety of activities. You need to have time for work, for family, for rest and relaxation and for personal interests. The secret ingredient is to make time for the things that are personally meaningful to you. These types of activities can be anything because they are unique to you. The skill is in knowing what it they are, carving out the time to do them and keeping them there as a priority to achieve and maintain personal wellbeing. Although this is not necessarily an easy process, making meaningful choices and having a sense of autonomy or control over workloads and life balance can help

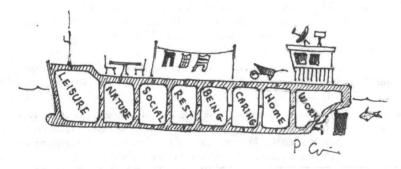

Figure 7.1 The Ship of Life
Adapted from Clouston (2015).

promote and maintain physical, mental, emotional and spiritual wellbeing while also ensuring that personal or family needs are not neglected (Mills & Chapman 2016, p. 88).

Step 2: Calming the mind

Thoughts are fascinating things: although we create them and are instrumental in how they influence our everyday psychological wellbeing, we often have very little apparent control over them. Sometimes they can be running wild in our minds, and we may not even be aware of them or of how much they are impacting on our wellbeing. Depending on your personality and circumstances at any one time, your thoughts can become very negative; you might find yourself ruminating and catastrophising about work or other aspects of life, and this can really affect how you feel.

If this is you, the first trick is to become aware of your thinking. Once you recognise you are worrying, you need to acknowledge that negative thoughts can frequently distort the facts, maybe by imagining the worst possible outcome. If you become conscious of this in your own pattern of thinking, then begin to revise it: reimagine it in a positive way and identify a more rational or evidence-based appraisal of events. Once you have done this, put the more positive and accurate pattern into action and commit to making the changes necessary to achieve that outcome (Clouston 2015). For example, if you find you are becoming enmeshed in work-based politics, then try to meaningfully detach yourself from them by making an active choice to change any negative thought patterns and reduce the intensity of your emotional and cognitive response to the situation (Devenish-Meares 2019). Nurture your personal attributes of coherence to help you here – motivation, a positive outlook, problem-solving and having a sense of control and autonomy will all help.

Step 3: Being present in the moment

Mindfulness has become a very popular practice to manage stress and anxiety. It is about living in the present moment as that moment unfolds, recognising thoughts as thoughts and finding the ability to be compassionate to both self and others (Neff 2003). Being present in the moment is a technique of pausing and intentionally paying attention in the here and now. People find this hard to do, and it can require some practice (Clouston 2015). However, if you can learn to be fully present in the moment, rather than multitasking or being focused on the next job, you can engage more meaningfully in whatever you are actually doing in a particular moment in time, become more self-aware and, through that focused process, experience a heightened sense of satisfaction and wellbeing. Through heightening awareness, mindfulness is believed to enhance your ability to practise self-care and compassion, and then, over time, to extend that ability to others, including in the workplace (Shapiro 2009, p. 556). This can then support a healthy work culture and experience, as well as reflecting the qualities and constructs of values-based leadership. It is easy to see how fostering Antonovsky's (1996) three dispositional traits could influence your abilities in practising mindfulness.

Step 4: Finding meaning in life

Meaning in life is often linked to the spiritual dimension of wellbeing: it is about 'being' who you want to be, having a sense of purpose and feeling fulfilled and satisfied with how you are living your life. When you have a sense of meaning in life you engage more, are more productive and your wellbeing improves (Clouston 2015). This fits directly with Antonovsky's (1996) notion of living with integrity and having a positive outlook, and means you are more effective and more satisfied as a person, both inside and outside of work.

However, in common with life balance, this construct is not easy to achieve in neoliberal societies unless paid work happens to be your meaningful activity, in which case you may be able to fulfil it without compromise. If this is you, great; but it's worth considering whether other activities in your life have been lost in the quest for success at work (think of your 'Ship of Life' here). If so, then is this an issue to address in terms of your personal wellbeing? Just give it some thought. Remember that strength and resilience can be found in diverse activities and a healthy work–life balance rather than a unilateral focus on one or two activities.

Finally, if your personal meaning is located in activities outside of work and you are compromising them, then you may find yourself feeling dissatisfied and unfulfilled because these are put aside to meet the demands of work activities. If this is you, then put your meaningful activities back into your life. Stop the compromise and reconcile your thinking to accept that having a little bit of time and energy for personal meaning in life can go a long way to nurturing your wellbeing.

Step 5: Self-knowledge, empowerment and integrity

As a leader, and indeed as a person, knowing yourself in terms of your own personal values and beliefs and your own moral compass is integral to wellbeing because these shape who you are and how you live or want to live your life. Self-knowledge is critical to understanding what is important to you as an individual and influences how you can sustain personal integrity and meaning in work and the rest of everyday life. Dissonance, or a lack of congruence between who you are and your workplace values or culture, can create disharmony. This is often manifest in ethical and moral dilemmas at a personal level and/or caused by differences between organisational demands and policies and the wants and needs of staff. (See Figure 9.1 for the 'Values Tree' exercise, which will help you scope your values and professional ethics.)

If this is an issue for you, then consider how the principles of values-based leadership might help. Centred on the constructs of trust, authenticity, integrity and equity (Wong & Walsh 2020), they are considered essential to create positive workplace cultures that promote wellbeing (Inceoglu et al. 2018; Wong & Cummings 2009) and reduce workplace bullying and burnout (Laschinger & Fida 2014). Theoretically, this approach requires you to support and empower staff to achieve organisational outcomes while also facilitating their progress to achieve their highest potential (Caldwell & Anderson 2020) – in the words of Denier et al. (2019, p. 1), giving them 'wings to fly'.

However, making choices that work for you, or your staff, can be difficult in the politics of power. My own work has shown that, although flexible working policies may be present for staff, accessing them in a meaningful way in pressured work environments can be challenging. This is because the major factor considered in the decision-making process is not personal choice to meet individual staff needs, but rather organisational requirements (Clouston 2015). If you find yourself in this kind of dilemma, then the interesting ethical framework in Figure 7.2 may just help you find a solution that meets both the organisational and the individual staff member's requirements. Developing Forsyth's (1980) well-known ethical ideology, Reiter (2007) applied his principles to addressing work–life balance dilemmas. In essence the framework provides a lens to consider how you can find a solution to satisfy a staff member's needs or wants in terms

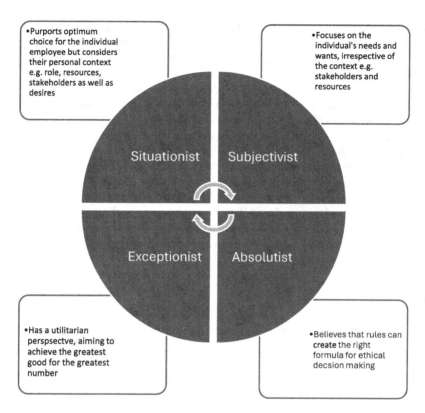

• Purports optimum choice for the individual employee but considers their personal context e.g. role, resources, stakeholders as well as desires

• Focuses on the individual's needs and wants, irrespective of the context e.g. stakeholders and resources

Situationist   Subjectivist

Exceptionist   Absolutist

• Has a utilitarian perspsectve, aiming to achieve the greatest good for the greatest number

• Believes that rules can create the right formula for ethical decsion making

Figure 7.2 Ethical framework for decision making

Adapted from Reiter (2007).

of, say, flexible working, and maintain the required human resources in the workplace. It is an interesting lens, and one I have found helpful in several different scenarios.

Let's consider the example of a request for four-day working. A staff member requires this to support personal wellbeing and childcare commitments on Mondays. As team leader you are aware that staffing is tight and there is pressure on the team; you are also aware that the staff member would benefit from dropping the day. You advocate and attempt to implement a values-based and compassionate approach to leadership within the constraints of your organisational setting; consequently, you find yourself in a bit of a quandary as to what to do. Looking at Figure 7.2, you begin to consider the different ways you could approach this issue.

Your first consideration is the 'subjectivist' view – i.e., what the individual needs is paramount. Now you want to support the staff member, and feel you should; you also consider them a friend, and this is heightening your awareness that you want to support them. However, if you make your decision based on this perspective or your personal preference, and you do not consider the rest of the team, the organisational pressures and the service users, you could fall into the trap of nepotism – or, at the very least, possible inequity in your decision making.

The 'absolutist' lens throws you back to the rules and asks you to consider what the right solution might be in this situation. As the existing post is full time and that is needed in the workplace, it suggests you should refuse the request. However, this offers you no option to support the staff member, who is struggling with personal wellbeing and home pressures. In a similar vein, the utilitarian 'exceptionist' perspective highlights the view that if you must achieve the greatest good for the majority, then you must again fall into refusing the request and maintain the status quo.

This brings you to the final perspective – the situationist view – which, like the subjectivist view, allows you to consider the needs of the staff member, but tempers that with the needs of the setting and its stakeholders. It requires you to consider both perspectives and review how you might be able to meet the staff member's request and maintain the organisational equilibrium: you are asked to contemplate 'Is there a workable solution?' In the end, you find that you can support the request if the staff member changes the day they want to drop to a less busy one for the service. They advise they can work with their present childcare provider to drop another day, allowing an acceptable and achievable outcome for both service and staff member. This may not be the ideal, but it is a satisfactory and manageable solution. Finally, if you are unclear on your own values and beliefs or are not sure where your moral compass is pointing, an online hub curated by Clouston et al. (2017) provides some great resources to help you explore and review this.

Reflective Activity: 7.3

Think about the five steps to improve wellbeing outlined above and how they resonate with you.

Write down your thoughts

Reflect on how you can make changes in your life to achieve a better sense of life balance and wellbeing.

7.6   CONCLUSION

So what have we learnt in our journey through this chapter? We set out to investigate the relationship between leadership and wellbeing, and questioned whether or not these two things were compatible. We found that, although there is liminality between the two and they are challenging to each other, there are ways forward to make them work together more effectively. First, as a leader, there are personal dispositions that you can hold or develop that can assist in facilitating and maintaining both your own and staff wellbeing. Antonovsky's (1996) notion of salutogenesis or a sense of personal coherence is one way to envisage the necessary qualities you need to attain in a personal context. It has also become clear that knowing who you are in terms of personal values and beliefs is an essential tool in wellbeing (Clouston 2015). When you are self-aware in this way, you can review whether or not this is reflective of who you are or aspire to be, and whether or not you need to do some work to address this.

Through self-awareness you can also establish how your preferred perspective 'fits' with your organisation's and whether or not it connects with the prism of values-based leadership. The latter is important because, in the landscape of wellbeing, a more values-based approach can offer a leadership framework that promotes wellbeing for all members of the organisation by engendering positive workplace cultures that genuinely value staff and nurture purpose, empowerment, integrity and choice.

Finally, we have explored techniques to support your own and others' wellbeing – i.e., living a balanced lifestyle, handling thoughts, living in the moment and finding meaning in life. Hopefully these will assist not only in your work but also in everyday life.

REFERENCES

Antonovsky, A. 1987. *Unravelling the mystery of health: How people manage stress and stay well.* San Francisco: Jossey-Bass.
Antonovsky, A. 1996. The salutogenic model as a theory to guide health promotion. *Health Promotion International,* 11(1), 11–18.
Bailey, S., & West, M. 2022. *What is compassionate leadership?* The King's Fund. https://www.kingsfund.org.uk/publications/what-is-compassionate-leadership#the-four-behaviours-of-compassionate-leadership [Accessed: 30 September 2022].
Caldwell, C., & Anderson, V. 2020. *Empowerment is a choice.* New York: Nova.
Clouston, T.J. 2014. Whose occupational balance is it anyway? The challenge of neoliberal capitalism and work–life imbalance. *British Journal of Occupational Therapy,* 77(10), 507–515.
Clouston, T.J. 2015. *Challenging stress, burnout and rust-out: Finding balance in busy lives.* London: Jessica Kingsley.
Clouston, T.J., Latham-Hastings, G., Paul-Taylor, G., Potton, R., & Ferriday, R. 2017. Becoming a caring & compassionate practitioner in health and social care practice. https://caringpractitioner.co.uk.
Coulthard, S., McGregor, J.A., & White, C. 2018. Multiple dimensions of wellbeing in practice. In: Schreckenberg, K., Mace, G., & Poudyal, M. (eds), *Ecosystem services and poverty alleviation.* London: Routledge, pp. 243–256.
Denier, Y., Dhaene, L., & Gastmans, C. 2019. 'You can give them wings to fly': A qualitative study on values-based leadership in health care. *BMC Medical Ethics,* 20, Art. 35. https://doi.org/10.1186/s12910-019-0374-x.
Devenish-Meares, P. 2019. Extending the heuristic inquiry research process to enable improved psycho-spiritual self-care choices associated with workplace stress and suffering. *International Journal of Academic Research in Business and Social Sciences,* 9(6), 866–889.
Eriksson, M., & Mittelmark, M.B. 2017. The sense of coherence and its measurement. In: Mittelmark, M.B. et al. (eds), *The handbook of salutogenesis.* New York: Springer, pp. 97–106.
Forsyth, D.R. 1980. A taxonomy of ethical ideologies. *Journal of Personality and Social Psychology,* 39, 175–184.
Galletta, M. et al. 2019. Sense of coherence and physical health-related quality of life in Italian chronic patients: The mediating role of the mental component. *BMJ Open,* 9(9). doi:10.1136/bmjopen-2019-030001 [Accessed: 26 February 2024].
Inceoglu, I., Thomas, G., Chu, C., Plans, D., & Gerbasi, A. 2018. Leadership behavior and employee wellbeing: An integrated review and a future research agenda. *Leadership Quarterly,* 29(1), 179–202. https://doi.org/10.1016/j.leaqua.2017.12.006.
Laschinger, H.K.S., & Fida, R. 2014. New nurses burnout and workplace wellbeing: The influence of authentic leadership and psychological capital. *Burnout Research,* 1(1), 19–28.
Mills, J., & Chapman, M. 2016. Compassion and self-compassion in medicine. *Australasian Medical Journal,* 9(5), 87–91.
Neff, K.D. 2003. Self-compassion: An alternative conceptualization of a healthy attitude toward oneself. *Self and Identity,* 2(2), 85–101.
Reiter, N. 2007. Work-life balance: What DO you mean? The ethical ideology underpinning appropriate application. *Journal of Applied Behavioural Science,* 43, 273–294.
Shapiro, S. 2009. The integration of mindfulness and psychology. *Journal of Clinical Psychology,* 65(6), 555–560.
Simons, G., & Baldwin, D.S. 2021. A critical review of the definition of well-being for doctors and their patients in a post COVID-19 era. *International Journal of Social Psychiatry,* 67(8), 984–2991.
Stanley, D. 2022. Clinical (values-based/congruent) leaders. In: Stanley, D., Bennett, C., & James, A.H. (eds), *Clinical leadership in nursing and healthcare.* Hoboken: Wiley, pp. 439–450.
Webb, P. 2023. Metaphors for wellbeing: Creating new metaphors. *M/C Journal,* 26(4). https://doi.org/10.5204/mcj.2979.
West, M. 2021. *Compassionate leadership: Sustaining humanity wisdom and presence in health and social care.* Swirling Leaf Press.
Wong, A.C., & Walsh, E.J. 2020. Reflections of a decade of authentic leadership in health care. *Journal of Nursing Management,* 28(1), 1–3. https://doi.org/10.1111/jonm.12861.
Wong, C.A., & Cummings, G.G. 2009. Authentic leadership: A new theory for nursing or back to basics? *Journal of Health Organization and Management,* 23(5), 522–538. https://doi.org/10.1108/14777260910984014.
World Health Organization. 2023. Promoting well-being. Available at: https://www.who.int/activities/promoting-well-being#:~:text=Well%2Dbeing%20encompasses%20quality%20of,sense%20of%20meaning%20and%20purpose [Accessed: 10 October 2023].

PART 2

INTRODUCTION TO PART 2
Methods and guides for developing personal leadership

The second part of this book presents some examples of methods, guides and exercises which you may find helpful in thinking about and developing your personal leadership. The following chapters offer some of the approaches available to developing leadership and can be applied at any time in the career. Some are helpful if used continually (such as journaling) or intermittently, revisited and combined to address different aspects of leadership advancement. Some will be helpful for you to reflect on and complete alone, such as the 'Values Tree' exercise in Chapter 9, whereas Chapter 11 on action learning aims to help you both support your facilitation skills and apply them within teams and groups to further problem solve.

Chapter 8 takes this forward by continuing the theme of emotional intelligence presented in Chapter 5, and expands to consider what it takes to become an emotionally intelligent professional, with scenario examples and reflective learning points. In Chapter 9 we explore the concept of professional and personal values, which we introduced in the first part of this book and discussed further in Chapter 2. Suggested exercises and methods of exploring values, ethics and what they mean for your leadership are offered. Chapter 10 takes us back to reflection and reflexivity, creativity and how creative methods such as journaling, visual thinking strategies and storytelling can support your leadership development over time. Chapter 11 presents Action Learning as a tool and technique for problem solving and developing personal skills such as facilitation. We hope you find these helpful for your continuing leadership journey.

DOI: 10.4324/9781003433354-9

CHAPTER 8

BECOMING A SELF-AWARE PROFESSIONAL
Developing emotional and social intelligence

Mandy Brimble

8.1 INTRODUCTION

The aim of this chapter is to: revisit the concepts of social and emotional intelligence outlined in Chapter 5; give an overview of how these skills can be developed; and use a case study to demonstrate how leaders can use social and emotional intelligence in challenging situations. Interactive activities will help the reader explore how leadership is underpinned by emotional and social intelligence skills at key points in 'Jenny's' career – from being a student to becoming an experienced practitioner. Alternative approaches to each situation are also considered.

8.2 DEVELOPING SOCIAL AND EMOTIONAL INTELLIGENCE SKILLS

Social and emotional intelligence are of increased importance in senior healthcare roles; but, clearly, they do not suddenly 'arrive' in the psyche when an individual progresses up the organisational ladder. Further, as shown by Mansel and Einion (2019) and Awwad et al. (2020) and discussed in Chapter 5, emotional intelligence skills can be eroded by the pressures of senior roles. So, it is important that social and emotional intelligence skills are nurtured throughout the healthcare career because they are not only important at every level but can also be developed incrementally over the career trajectory. Certain traits may require further development as roles change, so it is important for individuals to identify areas for development throughout their career. Although many social and emotional intelligence traits are intrinsic, they can also be learnt (Goleman 2020). Raising awareness of this skill set is the first step as many healthcare professionals do not fully understand it (Wilson 2014, Mansel & Einion 2019); hence the inclusion of these topics in this book.

Once basic knowledge and understanding of the concepts of social and emotional intelligence are in place, the next step is for the individual to undertake self-assessment. Examples of tools that enable self-assessment include: the Tromsø Social Intelligence Scale (TSIS), a self-report measure of social intelligence (Silvera et al. 2001); and the Mayer, Salovey, Caruso Emotional Intelligence Test (MSCEIT) (Mayer et al. 2002). However, due to the close relationship between social and emotional intelligence, it could be argued that such scales can assess competencies in both areas. For example, the Bar-On Emotional Quotient Inventory (Bar-On 2006) is designed to measure emotional and social strengths; but this is in the context of social skills being part of emotional intelligence rather than as a separate entity. More recently Shi et al. (2022) used existing scales to develop a validated social emotional skills scale. Whichever scale is used it is important that the same measures are used before and after developmental activities.

Formal training to develop social and emotional intelligence skills is available, and research shows that this can be effective (Schaap & Dippenaar 2017). However, these training courses can be expensive, time-consuming and not necessarily accessible to all. Foster et al. (2017) found that emotional intelligence skills developed incrementally in nursing students over the duration of the pre-registration programme, without any specific emotional intelligence

DOI: 10.4324/9781003433354-10

training. However, they state that this natural development of emotional intelligence should be enhanced by formal training within pre-registration curricula. Having said that, it is important to highlight that social and emotional intelligence skills can be developed on an independent individual basis, irrespective of career stage, by adopting the strategies outlined below.

Developing social intelligence

Joseph and Lakshmi (2010) state that knowing one's weaknesses and strengths is the starting point for developing social intelligence. Such knowledge could be gained from a self-assessment tool, as outlined above. They highlight skilled communication, empathy and team-building, problem-solving, decision-making and interaction skills as components of social intelligence. This list is helpful in highlighting the difference between social and emotional intelligence in that the latter is more about self-awareness, self-regulation and self-control, while the former is more about the ability to interact as part of a group.

Social intelligence can be developed with learning and practice by focusing on some key aspects of interpersonal interactions. Roshni (2023) highlights the following facets and provides guidance on how an individual can improve their skills in each area.

Pay close attention to what (and who) is around you

Socially intelligent people observe others and pay close attention to subtle social clues. Identify someone who has strong social skills, watch how they interact with others and model their behaviour.

Respect cultural differences

Go beyond this; seek learning to gain greater understanding. Most individuals learn social skills from their family, friends and community; but a socially intelligent person appreciates that others' responses may be different because of their customs and upbringing.

Practise active listening

- Don't interrupt.
- Take time to think about what has been said before you respond.
- Listen to inflections in speech as they can reveal the real meaning behind what is being said.

Appreciate the important people in your life

Pay attention to the emotions of your close family, friends, co-workers and peers. Ignoring cues from those closest to you hinders your ability to connect with them.

Work on increasing your emotional intelligence

Due to the close link between social and emotional intelligence there is a logical overlap in the development of these skills. Developing emotional intelligence is discussed in the following sub-section.

Developing emotional intelligence

In common with nurturing social intelligence skills, the development of emotional intelligence requires motivation, practice, listening to feedback and constant reinforcement of new skills (Serrat 2017, pp. 329–339). Herrity (2023) provides the following advice on self-development of emotional intelligence. You will note the inevitable commonalities with Roshni (2023) above.

Be more self-aware

Self-awareness is an essential skill that underpins many other emotional intelligence constructs (Goleman 1995). Tuning into your emotions and being aware of your emotional responses can improve emotional intelligence. When you feel a strong emotion, think about what caused you to feel that way. Improving self-awareness will help you process your emotions and communicate your feelings in a more measured manner.

Recognise how others feel

Although emotional intelligence starts with self-awareness, it is important to also gauge others' perceptions of your behaviour and communication. Adjusting ways of communicating and behaviours, based on cues from others, is a key component of emotional intelligence. However, these perceptions may not be obvious. If you are not sure about how others are feeling, ask them. This clearly demonstrates that you are prioritising them and respecting their feelings.

Practise active listening

Herrity (2023) highlights the importance of paying attention to non-verbal communication, so watch as well as listen for positive or negative reactions. Time taken to listen to others also indicates a level of respect, which is essential in healthy relationships. You can demonstrate active listening by asking questions and nodding. Repeating important points demonstrates that you have been listening and is important for checking you have understood what has been communicated.

Communicate clearly

Strong communication skills are key to emotional intelligence. Knowing how to say or write what you want to convey, and recognising the right time to do it, is critical for strong relationships. Try to be as communicative as you can (remembering to also listen – see above), and use multiple channels so others can easily communicate with you.

Stay positive

Be aware of the power of positive words, encouragement and kind gestures. Try to stay positive in stressful situations; it helps those around you remain calm and encourages problem-solving and teamwork. Negative emotions are normal, but try to minimise displaying these (note again the importance of self-awareness here) and focus on solutions rather than problems.

Empathise

As highlighted earlier, it is important to consider how others may be feeling. Doing so enables you to appreciate and understand these feelings (which may be different to your own) and respond in a respectful, comforting way. Empathy should be about considering how you might feel in another's situation, not about taking on the feelings of others as your own. (Refer back to Table 5.3 for types of empathy.)

Be open-minded

Try to be open to learning new things and embracing new ideas. It is natural to be wary of new things, but adopting an open-minded approach will mean that others will feel comfortable approaching you with their ideas. Never dismiss your own or others' ideas immediately because this stifles creativity and could mean that you miss problem-solving or personal/professional development opportunities.

Listen to feedback

Being open to both positive and negative feedback helps you take responsibility for your actions. Negative feedback can be challenging, but think of it as a positive; it is an opportunity to learn and grow both professionally and personally.

Remain calm under pressure

Approach stressful situations as calmly and positively as possible as it is easy for tension to escalate, particularly when there are deadlines or difficulties. Once again, focus on solutions rather than problems. Try to develop self-regulation strategies such as taking a deep breath, counting to ten or whatever has worked for you in the past. Don't be afraid to ask for help. From time to time, everyone will find themselves in a situation that they are unable to resolve alone.

8.3   USING SOCIAL AND EMOTIONAL INTELLIGENCE ACROSS THE CAREER LIFESPAN

This section will explore how 'Jenny', a fictitious nurse, uses social and emotional intelligence in challenging situations throughout her career.

Student nurse Jenny

Jenny is a student nurse about to start her first placement of year three. She is 24 years old and has a son aged five. Jenny worked as an insurance clerk before enrolling on the adult nursing degree programme. She is divorced but has good family support, with her parents, sister and ex-husband all contributing to childcare duties.

Just before starting the placement Jenny visited the ward to meet the staff and look around. She asked about requesting some specific days off in the third week of her placement. This was the first time in the programme that Jenny had to make any such request. The reason is that she has gaps in childcare provision due to her sister going on holiday. Jenny is told to write which days off she needs in the 'off-duty request book'. On her first shift Jenny is relieved to see that the rota shows she has been granted her requests. Jenny is nearing the end of her first week in placement. She goes on break with another member of staff. During their break her colleague tells Jenny that the ward manager was unimpressed by the number of requests Jenny had made, and that she should be available to work whenever needed. Jenny is shocked and upset. She wonders why the ward manager has discussed her grievance with other staff but not mentioned it to her, thus giving her the opportunity to explain. Jenny sees the ward manager when she returns to the ward but decides not to raise the issue straight away.

Jenny has a somewhat sleepless night worrying that she has made a bad impression. She also feels a little aggrieved as she has a good reason for needing the days off and has never made other requests. She also feels that the claim that she should be available to work whenever needed is unjustified due to the supernumerary status of nursing students. Jenny spends the next morning thinking about the situation. She reflects on what has been said about her, how that makes her feel, why the requests might be an issue for the ward manager, what she could have done to prevent the situation arising and what she should do now. Jenny thinks back to what has happened on previous placements and realises that she has had opportunities to self-roster providing certain conditions were met. That afternoon Jenny phones the ward and asks the manager if they could meet for a short while the following day. The ward manager asks what the meeting is about and pushes Jenny to speak about it there and then. Jenny politely says that she would rather discuss it in person.

When Jenny arrives for the meeting the next day the ward manager is a little off-hand and says, 'What's all the fuss about? Why couldn't we talk about this on the phone?' Jenny can feel herself blush and is conscious that her heart is racing. She takes a deep breath and thanks the ward manager for agreeing to meet with her. She says that she is afraid she has unintentionally created a bad impression and that she would like to rectify this. Jenny says she has been told that the ward manager is unhappy about her requests for time off. The manager nods. Jenny explains her domestic situation, the reason for the requests and that this is the first time in the programme that she has made requests. The ward manager seems a little taken aback to be approached directly about this but listens to what Jenny has to say. Jenny goes on to say that she now realises it would have been better to explain her situation at the outset rather than just putting the requests in the book as she was directed to.

The ward manager asks a few questions about Jenny's son and how she has managed so far. She then asks how she is going to manage when she is qualified. Jenny explains that, due to students' supernumerary status, some of the other areas of the programme have allowed her to self-roster (providing she was working with her practice supervisor or assessor for most shifts). She tells the ward manager that she intends to work part time when she is qualified and that, had there been an option to study the nursing programme part time she would have done so. Jenny thanks the ward manager again for her time and they part on amicable terms.

Reflective Activity: 8.1

Which aspects of social and emotional intelligence has Jenny demonstrated?

How did taking time to reflect contribute to how Jenny managed the situation?

What would Jenny have done differently if she had not been acting in a socially and emotionally intelligent way?

Would that have affected the outcome?

Could Jenny have done anything differently?

It is likely that you identified that Jenny demonstrated self-awareness and self-regulation when she decided not to approach the ward manager when she returned to the ward after her break. She used the time off between shifts to reflect on what had happened, how she felt and why. She also thought about why the requests may have been an issue for the ward manager, thereby demonstrating a desire to be empathetic. Jenny could have just let the situation rumble on (she had been granted her requests after all) but she chose to speak with the ward manager face to face, in a non-confrontational way. She demonstrated self-control when she felt challenged by the ward manager at the start of the meeting, and recognised that she was having a physical response to this. She used deep breathing to regulate her heart rate and reduce anxiety. She also took the opportunity to tactfully remind the ward manager that students are supernumerary. Describing the situation in terms of what a third party does, rather than pointing out what the individual involved should be doing, is a useful tactic when you want to make a point without being confrontational.

Staff nurse Jenny

Jenny has now been qualified for five years, and has been a Band 6 staff nurse on a surgical ward for the last year. She has remarried and feels settled in her personal life. Jenny is at the start of a day shift and is working with a second-year student, for whom she is practice supervisor. Jenny and the student are completing a pre-op checklist for 'George', who is due to have long-awaited surgery. Jenny is called away to the telephone and George tells the student he is worried that his surgery may be cancelled again. He explains that it had already been cancelled once due to lack of intensive therapy unit (ITU) beds. Jenny returns after finishing her phone call and they move on to another patient. Later, when they are alone, Jenny tells the student that the phone call was from George's son, who was quite verbally aggressive, saying that they had better not cancel the operation again and that, if they did, he would be coming in to 'sort them out'. Jenny notices that the student becomes wide-eyed and seems quite alarmed at what she has said. She reassures her that it is probably 'all bluster', but says that she will communicate this to other staff during handover.

George's surgery goes ahead as planned and is successful. Two days later George is transferred from the high dependency unit (HDU) to the ward. Jenny and the student are on a night shift. During handover it is mentioned that George had a visit from his son in the afternoon. The staff nurse who had been looking after George says that his son did not visit for long, seemed to be in a rush and was a little abrupt when he spoke to his father. Jenny and the student request that George be allocated to them as they have cared for him previously. It is a fairly quiet shift. George wakes during the night, so Jenny and the student spend some time speaking with him. George asks when he will be discharged. Jenny reassures him that it will be soon. George says, 'Oh that's good', but Jenny and the student notice that his facial expression is not in keeping with his words, and that he is showing signs of agitation, tapping his fingers, clenching his fists and jiggling his legs. Jenny offers to make George a cup of tea, which he accepts. Both Jenny and the student go to the kitchen to make the tea.

Jenny is thinking about what just happened. She wonders why George might be agitated about being discharged. Initially, based on his son's behaviour, she thinks that perhaps he is not very kind to George. The student is very agitated, saying that she learnt about 'elder abuse' at university and, based on the verbal aggression displayed by George's son, she thinks this is why George doesn't want to go home. She asks Jenny if the day staff should be told to phone the Adult Safeguarding Team at Social Services. Jenny tells the student that they must keep an open mind and would need much more information before taking any action. She says she hopes that sharing a hot drink with George will encourage him to reveal why his recent words and body language are contradictory.

Jenny, the student and George drink their tea and chat about inconsequential matters. Just as they are finishing and Jenny moves to get up, George grasps her arm and says, 'Please stay for a little longer.' Jenny and the student sit down, and Jenny asks George if there is anything he would like to tell her. George is silent for a while, but Jenny resists the urge to fill the silence or tell George she needs to get on with her work. Jenny uses non-verbal body language to communicate that the student should also remain quiet. George eventually tells them that he is lonely and is not looking forward to going home as he has enjoyed the company of other patients and staff. He explains that he moved house three years earlier to be nearer his son and his family, leaving behind friends and the village he had lived in for years. However the move has not worked out as expected. George thought he would see his son, his daughter-in-law and his grandchildren regularly, but his son is busy with his job and his wife always seems to be taking the children to sports practice or other activities. George only sees them about once a month. George explains that his son has a 'short fuse' and becomes exasperated when George asks when he will see him and the grandchildren.

George wants to make the best of the situation, even though he feels let down by his son. He has joined clubs in the area, but it has been difficult to make new friends. Recently his ill-health has prevented him attending the clubs, but he is hoping that when he recovers from surgery he will be able to start attending again. Jenny encourages George to do this. She also offers to speak with George's son, but George doesn't want this. He says he will try to speak with his daughter-in-law to ask if perhaps he could accompany her when she takes the children to their sporting activities.

Reflective Activity: 8.2

Which aspects of social and emotional intelligence has Jenny demonstrated?

What would Jenny have done differently if she had not been acting in a socially and emotionally intelligent way?

Would that have affected the outcome?

Could Jenny have done anything differently?

Hopefully you identified that Jenny demonstrated leadership alongside social and emotional intelligence when she shared information, about the telephone call from George's son, with the student in private. This would have demonstrated leadership in terms of keeping information confidential together with avoiding escalation of anxiety in other staff. Jenny did, of course, safeguard other staff by sharing this information in the privacy of handover.

Jenny also demonstrated socially and emotionally intelligent leadership by reading George's body language and recognising that it contradicted what he was saying. The student also demonstrated these skills, but she jumped to conclusions about what this meant. Experience, taking time to reflect and following Jenny's role-modelling should help the student avoid this in the future. Jenny gave George the time and space to reveal the reason for his anxiety about returning home. Silence was very important here, and Jenny ensured that this was maintained by using body language to communicate this to the student, once again role modelling emotional and social intelligence.

Had Jenny acted differently – for example by ignoring George's cues, not keeping an open mind or by filling the silence because it felt awkward – there could have been dire consequences for George's son, even if any accusations were found to be false. This could also have damaged the already fragile relationship between George and his son. In terms of her relationship with George, Jenny would have failed to uncover the real reason for his anxiety, leaving him feeling unimportant and unsupported. Fundamentally, there may not be anything Jenny could do to improve George's situation; but sometimes just being receptive, helping someone feel heard and taking time to listen can make a significant difference to how they feel about themselves.

Jenny the Directorate Manager

Jenny has now been qualified for 15 years and is the Directorate Manager for surgical nursing at a large hospital. The COVID-19 pandemic started two months ago, so only essential and emergency surgeries were going ahead. Although fewer surgeries are taking place, Jenny's workload is virtually the same due to overseeing personal protective equipment (PPE) requirements and other infection control matters. Resources, including staff, have been re-deployed to areas where patients with COVID are being cared for. Jenny had to manage this as most staff in line management positions were also being re-deployed, and therefore not available to organise their own staff. The re-deployments took place very swiftly, and Jenny still feels like her head is reeling from organising something so vast and important in such a short space of time. She worries about whether she did a good job; and, even though she arrives home exhausted, she is unable to sleep at night. Jenny is hopeful that the staff she is overseeing are embracing challenges and opportunities for learning new skills, but fears that some may be unhappy. This is one of the things that keep her awake at night. However, she has avoided delving into this too deeply as she knows she does not have much control over the re-deployments now they are in place.

Four months into the pandemic Jenny meets a colleague, Sarah, in the car park. She is leaving for home and Sarah is arriving for work. Sarah was previously a ward manager on the children's surgical ward but has been re-deployed to an adult HDU. Jenny greets Sarah warmly; they have worked together for many years and were, in fact, in the same cohort during their nurse training, albeit studying different fields of nursing. Sarah does not reciprocate Jenny's greeting and looks away when Jenny starts to talk to her. Jenny is a little shocked by Sarah's 'cool' response and asks if there is anything the matter. Sarah responds with a tirade of loud, angry words. She says that Jenny has 'thrown her under the bus' in assigning her to the adult HDU. She reminds Jenny that she is a children's nurse and, apart from one adult surgical ward placement during her training, has never worked in adult care. Sarah states that she has been totally humiliated by having to ask junior nurses questions about nursing care. She says that if Sarah had given the situation any thought she would have moved another member of staff to the adult HDU and allowed her to remain in charge of the children's surgeries that were going ahead. Before Jenny can respond Sarah rushes off. Jenny is really shaken by the encounter and wonders how many other members of her staff feel the same. She is tempted to catch up with Sarah but realises that it is probably better not to approach her while she is so angry.

Having given the encounter some thought, Jenny contacts Sarah and suggests they meet on an off-duty day and go for a socially distanced walk (as per COVID restrictions). Sarah is resistant at first but eventually agrees. Initially Jenny keeps the conversation to neutral topics to break the ice. She starts the conversation about the work issue by being transparent, stating that she has been worried about decisions made in relation to re-deployment. She says she understands why Sarah is upset and that she appreciates how difficult it would be to defer to junior colleagues when she has been accustomed to using her knowledge and expertise to support and direct others. Sarah apologises for her outburst the previous week and says she should have arranged to meet Jenny at work to talk about her grievance. She states that having to defer to junior colleagues is not really the issue; it is more about the distress she has experienced while caring for patients with COVID-19 due to being unsure about whether she is giving the best possible standard of care. She says that she also had an argument with one of her teenage sons on the day she bumped into Jenny, so she was still angry about that when they met.

Jenny thanks Sarah for the explanation and clarifying what the main issue is. They talk this through, and Jenny asks Sarah to explain why she thinks she may have not given the best possible care to her patients. Jenny listens carefully, nodding to indicate that she is being attentive to what Sarah is saying and does not interrupt. Jenny states that she can appreciate Sarah feels she has not maintained her usual exceptionally high standards. She reassures her that feedback from the HDU manager has been really positive, and highlights that she has cared for a different patient group under very difficult circumstances to the best of her ability. Jenny chooses her words and tone carefully to ensure that she does not patronise Sarah but gets her point across. Jenny tells Sarah she may not be able to change things for her, but asks: 'In an ideal world what would you want to happen?' Sarah pauses to think and says that, although she has struggled with working in the adult HDU, she couldn't possibly consider abandoning her patients.

Reflective Activity: 8.3

Which aspects of social and emotional intelligence has Jenny demonstrated?

What would Jenny have done differently if she had not been acting in a socially and emotionally intelligent way?

Would that have affected the outcome?

Could Jenny have done anything differently?

Hopefully you will have spotted that Jenny behaved in a socially and emotionally intelligent way by not trying to pursue the conversation with Sarah during their initial encounter. She took time to reflect and to give Sarah space. When they met later, she was open and transparent with Sarah. She gave Sarah the opportunity to 'offload' and made it clear she was listening. She helped Sarah identify the main issue and was honest about how much she could do to change the situation. This helped Sarah reconnect with her core caring values and motivations. Had Jenny been defensive at any point in the initial encounter, pushed Sarah to speak with her when she was angry or made unrealistic promises that she could not fulfil, this situation could have deteriorated.

In terms of what Jenny could have done differently, she could have set aside time to meet, face to face or online, with the re-deployed ward managers to check on how they were coping in their new areas. She could have asked them to link in with their previous direct reports to check on their wellbeing. This would have facilitated a check-in by a familiar person and complemented any support they were already receiving in their new areas.

8.4   CONCLUSION

This chapter has outlined strategies for self-development of social and emotional intelligence skills. Socially and emotionally intelligent leadership is illustrated by an in-depth exploration of key events in the career of a fictitious nurse named Jenny. The reader was invited, via interactive activities, to consider Jenny's approach in each situation. These activities were followed by an expert narrative designed to promote understanding of the relevant social and emotional intelligence concepts under consideration. Alternative approaches to the situations were also considered.

REFERENCES

Awwad, D.A., Lewis, S.J., Mackay, S., & Robinson, J. 2020. Examining the relationship between emotional intelligence, leadership attributes and workplace experience of Australian chief radiographers. *Journal of Medical Imaging and Radiation Sciences*, 51(2), 256–263.

Bar-On, R. 2006. The Bar-On model of emotional-social intelligence (ESI). *Psicothema*, 18(Supplement), 13–25. https://www.psicothema.com/pdf/3271.pdf.

Foster, K., Fethney, J., McKenzie, H., Fisher, M., Harkness, E., & Kozlowski, D. 2017. Emotional intelligence increases over time: A longitudinal study of Australian pre-registration nursing students. *Nurse Education Today*, 55, 65–70.

Goleman, D. 1995. *Emotional intelligence: Why it can matter more than IQ.* New York: Bantam.

Goleman, D. 2020. *Emotional intelligence: Why it can matter more than IQ.* 25th anniversary edition. London: Bloomsbury.

Herrity, J. 2023. How to improve emotional intelligence in 9 steps. https://www.indeed.com/career-advice/career-development/how-to-improve-emotional-intelligence [Accessed: 28 January 2024].

Joseph, C. & Lakshmi, S.S. 2010. Social intelligence, a key to success. *IUP Journal of Soft Skills*, 4(3), 15–21.

Mansel, B. and Einion, A. 2019. 'It's the relationship you develop with them': Emotional intelligence in nurse leadership. A qualitative study. *British Journal of Nursing* 28(21), pp. 1400–1408. doi:10.12968/bjon.2019.28.21.1400.

Mayer, J.D., Salovey, P., & Caruso, D.R. (2002). *Mayer-Salovey-Caruso emotional intelligence test (MSCEIT) users manual.* Toronto, ON: Multi-Health Systems (MHS). https://scholars.unh.edu/personality_lab/27/ [Accessed: 21 January 2024].

Roshni, M.J. 2023. Social intelligence. https://www.linkedin.com/pulse/social-intelligence-roshni-m-j/ [Accessed: 28 January 2024].

Schaap, P. & Dippenaar, M. 2017. The impact of coaching on the emotional and social intelligence competencies of leaders. *South African Journal of Economic and Management Sciences*, 20(1). doi:10.4102/sajems.v20i1.1460.

Serrat, O. 2017. *Knowledge solutions: Tools, methods, and approaches to drive organizational performance.* Singapore: Springer.

Shi, J., Cheung, A.C.K., Zhang, W. & Tam, W.W.Y. 2022. Development and validation of a social emotional skills scale: Evidence of its reliability and validity in China. *International Journal of Educational Research*, 114(4), 102007. doi:10.1016/j.ijer.2022.102007.

Silvera, D.H., Martinussen, M., & Dahl, T.I. 2001. The Tromsø Social Intelligence Scale, a self-report measure of social intelligence. *Scandinavian Journal of Psychology*, 42(3), 313–319.

Wilson, J. 2014. The awareness of emotional intelligence by nurses and support workers in an acute hospital setting. *Journal of Health Sciences*, 2(9), 458–464.

CHAPTER 9

EXPLORING PERSONAL VALUES FOR LEADERSHIP

Alison H. James

9.1 INTRODUCTION

In the first part of this book we explored values and why they are important in leadership development. Identifying your values and what is important to you, on both a personal and a professional level, can provide insights into what kind of leader you want to be. Being clear about your own values can also provide you with direction in determining what profession(s) these align with and what career path is right for you. This applies to all levels of positional and personal leadership, so these exercises can be applicable at any stage in your career and at whatever positional level you are practising. Once you have chosen a path, it is also important to think about the organisation you work in and whether both your personal and professional values align with those the organisation sets out. Sometimes, if these three areas are not aligned, we find ourselves becoming dissatisfied with our work, career and professions, so checking back in with your values every now and then to see how they 'fit' with the other two areas, and vice versa, is a good habit to adopt in your leadership practice and career.

Leadership is a challenging passage and, because we are human, we may become distracted from our values base by demands or attractive, sometimes easier, power facets such as reward and acclaim or influencing individuals or cultures, or by needs such as social acceptance and wanting to be part of something. What we need to realise is that changing direction or making mistakes is human and, while we may stray, these are important learning opportunities and we can find our way back to our original aims. This is part of your emotional intelligence development as well as your self-awareness insight. Identifying your weaknesses is also part of this so you can have forewarning of areas you may be more vulnerable to. What is important is that we recognise these distractions and maintain focus, avoiding the pull towards sometimes easier yet potentially destructive routes.

In the Values Tree exercise in Reflective Activity 9.1, adapted from coaching techniques and models, you can begin to plot your values and think about how these align to your organisation. If you are interested in reading further about how these techniques can support decision making and exploring more detailed approaches, see Anderson (2002); and, for advancing towards future planning for setting goals and objectives, O'Neill (2000). You can revisit this exercise as your leadership and career progresses. Although your values may change over time, it is good to check how they align with your leadership goals and professional aims, along with reflecting on how you demonstrate these to others and why they are important to you.

Reflective Activity: 9.1

Images can help us reflect and visually plot out an issue, and here I have used a tree as an example (Figure 9.1). Draw your own image or use the one shown. Label the leaves on the tree with your values, which could be personal and/or professional, or draw two trees and plot these separately – although I would anticipate there will overlaps if you are in the right profession.

DOI: 10.4324/9781003433354-11

You will see in Figure 9.1 that the roots are labelled with areas concerned with ethics, so these will be the professional codes of practice that anchor your professional standards to your practice. In this example I have used the standards from the UK's Nursing and Midwifery Council (2018), but you can replace these with your own professional standards. These codes and standards, as with the roots of a tree, are essential and static, so they will not change; rather, they firmly establish what is acceptable, what is right and what is expected of you as a professional. To help you set out your values, think about the following:

- What is important to you?
- What makes you happy and fulfilled as an individual and as part of your profession?
- What values do you convey as part of your professional practice, for example, compassion, empathy?
- What makes you proud in your personal and professional life, and how do you convey this to others?
- What values would you like others to see in you?

Once you have identified your values, choose the five that are most important to you. This may require deeper thought as you will need to consider personal and professional priorities. When you have chosen your five core values, think about how they align to your personal and professional life. Reflect on how you demonstrate these values in your leadership approach. Are they clearly visible to others, and how can you make them clearer in your decision making, communication and teamwork?

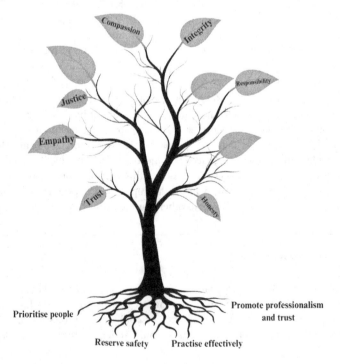

Figure 9.1 Values Tree exercise

9.2 VALUES IN PRACTICE

From the Values Tree exercise you will have reflected on what your values are and how you display these to others. In terms of your leadership practice this can cause moral dilemmas and challenges, as discussed in Chapter 2. For most day-to-day experiences you will be able to clearly exhibit your values in your decision making, in your communication with others and through your attentiveness and listening skills. However, when challenges occur, they can unbalance you, so it is good to have some techniques that will stabilise thinking and help you navigate the difficulties. Some useful techniques for wellbeing are set out in Chapter 7, and here we present some key questions to ask yourself if you feel challenged and unsure that your leadership is remaining values-focused.

Reflective Activity: 9.2

Think about a situation that was challenging to lead, for example: a time when your decisions were being questioned; you were asked to implement something you felt was not good for the area or team; a colleague was being challenging; or you were managing a conflict within your team.

Write down the scenario and reflect on what made it challenging for you to maintain your values. Which values in particular did you feel were difficult to maintain, and why? On reflection, do you feel you were able to maintain your values? If so, how did you overcome this difficulty? Did you seek feedback on how you led the situation?

Now think about the following tips and questions you can use in the future, which may help you through challenges to your values. Because decisions are sometimes made without time to truly reflect, opportunities to seek support and look ahead can be missed. By considering these and applying them to a past experience it is possible to learn from experience and be equipped with questions to seek solutions in advance of challenges in the future.

- Which core value or values are being challenged by this situation?
- Are ethical standards and codes being challenged in this situation?
- If someone else was describing this scenario, how would I advise them to navigate this?
- Am I able to negotiate a different action or approach to this?
- If I compromise my values, what might the consequences be for me, for the team, for others?
- Tomorrow, will I be content with the actions I chose to take?
- How can I seek support on this?
- Can I discuss this with a mentor or trusted colleague?

Moving forward from the challenges, it is also important to consider and amplify what you think you are good at or what your strengths are. You may be able identify some of these from the previous exercise. If you felt proud of the way you navigated your way through a challenging situation, this can be a powerful confirmation that you are developing as a leader and that you are maintaining your core values in that achievement. For the next set of exercises, consider your strengths and areas you feel need further development. By reflecting on these you can begin to write your leadership narrative and establish where you are and where you need to go.

Think about the skills needed to be an effective leader. Some of these are presented in Part 1 of this book, but you may want to consider others. Starting with the following set of exercises, adapted from Northouse (2012), reflect on what your strengths are. Then consider the areas you feel you can develop further and what, who or how you need to achieve this. This will be the start of your leadership narrative, unique to you, and which you can steer taking your leadership mastery forward.

Reflective Activity: 9.3a

An effective leader connects and communicates well with others, motivates others, allows others to express their ideas and flourish in their work environment.

- How well do you think you communicate with all staff?
- How do you support others in their development?
- How do you motivate others?
- How well do you work within a team?

Reflective Activity: 9.3b

Leading in your profession requires levels of knowledge and expertise in your area.

- Do you feel knowledgeable in your area of practice?
- What areas of knowledge would you like to explore, and how will this improve your practice?
- How can you seek further knowledge and development? What resources might you need and how can you gain these?
- Do you have a mentor?
- Can you access coaching?
- How well do you know your organisation?
- Where can you gain further insight into the organisation and how it functions?

Reflective Activity: 9.3c

Leaders work effectively with colleagues and peers at all levels. To do this requires self-awareness, emotional intelligence, social awareness and insight into the people you work with and the culture and organisation you work in.

- Do you understand what is important to others in your team?
- What are the main challenges for your team at the moment?

- How well do people respond to change and innovation?
- How are change and innovation encouraged, and do you motivate people in these areas?
- How well do you understand your own and others' emotions?
- How well do you facilitate emotions in your thinking?
- How well do you reason and understand your emotions?
- How would you describe the culture of your organisation?
- Do you confront issues of conflict or negativity?
- Can you deal with conflict effectively?

Reflective Activity: 9.3d

Effective leaders have good conceptual skills –for example, in problem solving, planning or creating a vision.

- How well do you identify problems, seek solutions and apply solutions?
- Are there techniques or tools you think you need to access to improve those skills?
- How well do you learn and find new information? How do you keep up to date with your area of expertise? Do you seek new evidence, and how do you apply it?
- How often do you use reflection and reflexivity in practice?
- How do you convey your vision to others?
- How do you engage with others to help you achieve your vision?

9.3 CONCLUSION

Leadership can be highly complex and challenging; however, you have established your core values and reflected on how these align with your professional and organisational values. You have considered areas of learning from past experience. You have also identified areas of strength in your leadership and areas where you can improve, and you have begun to think about how you can achieve this. Taking these methods forward, use them to set yourself goals, realise how far you have come and remind yourself of your potential to impact your profession.

REFERENCES

Anderson, B. 2002. *The three secrets of wise decision making*. Portland, OR: Single Reef Press.

Northouse, P.G. 2012. *Introduction to leadership: Concepts and practice*. 2nd edn. Thousand Oaks, CA: Sage.

Nursing and Midwifery Council. 2018. *The Code: Professional standards of practice and behaviour for nurses, midwives and nursing associates*. https://www.nmc.org.uk/globalassets/sitedocuments/nmc-publications/nmc-code.pdf [Accessed: 1 September 2024].

O'Neill, J. 2000. Smart goals, smart schools. *Educational Leadership*, 57(5), 46–50.

CHAPTER 10

CREATIVE METHODS FOR LEADERSHIP DEVELOPMENT

Alison H. James

10.1   INTRODUCTION

In Chapter 4 we looked at John Dewey's theories of learning and reflection, but he was also interested in the aesthetic experience and its impact on learning, the arts and how we can use these to reflect and think on a deeper level. In this context Dewey (1980) considered aesthetic experiences and the exploration of metaphors as helpful to stimulate thinking and allow associations to be made in thinking. Indeed, he views the aesthetic experience as reflecting the very nature of experience at a high level of knowledge. Here we apply this to the topic of leadership and how you can use different creative methods to support your thinking and development as a leader in your own context and to whatever level you choose. These methods are therefore useful throughout the career, and you may return to them on occasion to stimulate your perceptions, revisit experiences, reflect on those and build as your experience as a leader also develops. While you may think this requires much introspection, and these approaches can be effective for that, I am not advising navel-gazing. However, it is important for leaders to be self-aware, able to see progress in their leadership and to revisit their values and skills at various points in their career. Leaders need to be willing to analyse themselves and be transparent with others to be effective (Ford et al. 2008).

In teaching leadership and quality improvement I have used visual images, metaphors and symbolism for many years. I have found that students engage with the process and often express how they can dip into the 'toolbox' of methods as they progress. The methods explored here include visual thinking strategies, and there are some exercises to start you on your path to exploring this approach. Journaling is another helpful method of documenting your thoughts, reflecting on experiences and planning your leadership path. Finally, we will consider story-telling as a way of creating your own leadership development narrative and influencing and supporting others.

There are many other forms of creative learning of course, and they may make you think about how else you can develop them. It might be that you prefer much firmer constructive methods of learning, so the final chapter on action learning may be helpful if you are far more practical and structured in your approach. However, I would encourage you to try the methods outlined here; as reflective professionals, they should be familiar to your approach to learning and will helpfully allow you to further explore the possibilities.

10.2   WHAT HAS CREATIVITY TO DO WITH LEADERSHIP?

Although we may not associate creativity with many healthcare professions and healthcare education, it is present in areas such as occupational health. The focus instead tends to be on processes and techniques, science and procedural requirements, with little room for creative thinking and innovation. However this is changing somewhat as we acknowledge the need for quality improvement and innovation to address some of the challenges in healthcare and to enhance safety for patients. Nursing has been described as both an art and a science, although

DOI: 10.4324/9781003433354-12

that debate continues. We are all required to solve problems and be inquisitive, which is why we now base our practice on evidence, and healthcare has advanced dramatically over the last few centuries. It could be argued that most healthcare professionals are creative every day as we work in complex organisations and deal in the care of humankind – a context that is unpredictable and so requires adaptability and continual change.

Leadership education scholars recognise the need for imaginative pedagogies to support creativity in the development of leadership (Cranston & Kusanovich 2014, Klein 1998). If we consider the use of imagery, symbolism and metaphors in leadership, there are some large organisations and businesses that have become adept at using imagery to convey their values and philosophies. Think of Apple, founded in 1976 by Steve Jobs and Steve Wozniak, whose apple logo with a bite has become synonymous with its founders' productivity and effective leadership. Although it has evolved over time, the image is familiar and well known; although simplistic, it is effective. If you consider what you associate this image with, you might think of Isaac Newton and discovery, knowledge and abundance, along with substance and productivity, success and many others. A simple image can therefore be powerful and mean different things to different people.

With an increase in the use of digital images and alignment with aesthetics, artistic metaphors of leadership are being used to support leadership development and philosophies (Klenke 2016). To engage the creative imagination and passion associated with aesthetics – to create connections through metaphors – major corporations have employed artists and poets to enhance their employees' and customers' commitment (Klenke 2016, James 2020). Leadership theories have also used visual associations such as 'bridge-building leadership' within the complexity, cross-cultural theories of Stacey (2010).

Reflective Activity: 10.1

Let us consider what creativity can offer leadership development and how they are connected. I offer the following examples. Think about how they are similar and connected. You may disagree or you may think of others:

- Art, poetry and the written word can invoke emotion, can be stimulating and visionary. Leadership can also have this effect.
- Thinking about things differently can help solve problems, develop new insights and lead to innovation. Both creative arts and leadership are driven by these approaches.
- Leadership and creative art require time, practice and skill.
- Leadership and art are methods of communication and can influence, be inspiring and change the way we think.
- Both art and leadership require courage and commitment, can be accepting of failure and apply reflection, learn and start again.

Can you think of other ways creativity and leadership are similar or connected?

Stanley (2022) states that it is part of a leader's role to encourage an environment of innovation and enable others to express creativity. Effective leaders do not just understand individual meanings and perspectives; they also require the capacity to step back and observe a broad landscape. So, as leaders, we should accept the creative process as an advantage and opportunity. I would suggest it is also the role of leaders to be creative in their approach to self-development, to be courageous enough to explore their deeper thinking, applying methods they feel they may not wish to reveal to others, such as drawing or writing; yet this can be effective as a personal outlet for their creative learning.

10.3   IMAGES FOR LEADERSHIP

In my qualitative research of nursing students and academics, I used a narrative inquiry approach and photographic imagery to encourage reflection and association with leadership (James et al. 2022). The use of images in research can be effective to gain knowledge beyond analysis of an image itself as they enable interpretation according to views, experiences and values, providing a deeper exploration of symbolic reasoning (Collier & Collier 1986). Images can stimulate conversations in a group, and I explore the use of visual thinking strategies for learning in Section 10.4. On an individual level, using images to reflect, to think on a deeper level, to make associations and arrive at new ideas can be a powerful way to support your approach to leadership. Images can be a catalyst; they can invoke the memory of an event or be suggestive, stimulating emotions of that memory in a similar way that music, or the smell of something, can. You might look at an image that is pleasing; you may be drawn to the content, to the topic, to the colours.

Images work on many levels; and if we allow ourselves time to reflect, question and contemplate, they can help us arrive at new perceptions, new realisations and new ways of thinking. In my research I used images such as the moon reflected in the sea, which some participants thought represented power, the influence of gravitational force on the tide and waves and the reflection as influencing its followers, while the sea was the organisation as a collective mass and force (James 2020). Images of trees and roots were associated with protection, support, anchoring. While some participants initially looked at and described the images, when asked to think how they might be associated with leadership, further and more in-depth associations were formed and expressed, some evoking memories of events and experiences of leadership that led to reflective thoughts (James et al. 2022).

Reflective Activity: 10.2

Consider Figures 10.1–10.4. Look carefully at each image and consider the following questions. Write down your answers:

- What do you see in these images?
- Choose an image that reflects how you feel as a leader.
- What is it about this image that makes you associate it with your leadership development? Write down as much detail as possible.
- Now consider what your perspective on leadership was three years ago. Would you have chosen this picture then? If so, why and if not, why not?
- Now consider where you would like to be in three years' time. What do you hope to have improved on in terms of leadership? Would you still choose this image?
- Reflect on why you chose this image and what learning you can take forward. How far have you come in your leadership development? Can this be symbolised by this image?

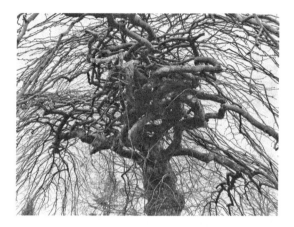

Figure 10.1 Tangled tree

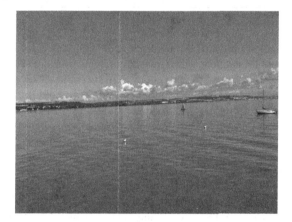

Figure 10.2 View across a bay

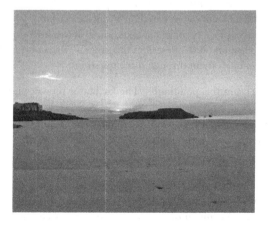

Figure 10.3 Sunrise

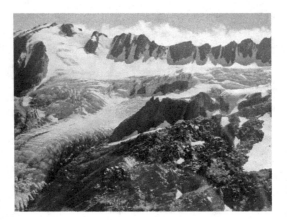

Figure 10.4 Glacier

You can use images like these to also think about different aspects of your work or career. For example, you could think about which image represents your organisation or your team, and apply the same type of questions and reflection. You could also ask someone else to give their thoughts and compare and contrast your views and perceptions. Images can work on an individual basis (for self-reflection) or within groups and teams to consider how well teams are working together or how they perceive their organisations. What is important is to move thinking forward, to challenge initial thoughts towards solving an issue or setting new goals and aims.

10.4   VISUAL THINKING STRATEGIES

'Visual Thinking Strategies' (VTS) is a teaching method which has been found to increase communication skills and observational skills, increase empathy and support reflection on experience (Moorman et al. 2016). This method, developed by Housen (2002), usually requires a visit to an art gallery and a facilitator, as based on Vygotsky's (1993 [1978]) social development theory – that learning takes place in social contexts; and this can help students develop connections in their learning. Housen (2002) describes the process whereby a facilitator asks students to look at a painting and takes them through three questions:

- What is going on in this painting? – The facilitator repeats and affirms the students' response.
- What are you seeing that makes you say that? – This requires the students to revisit the image and evidence their thoughts.
- What more can we find? – This encourages the students to find deeper meaning.

All contributions are valued equally.

In their work on VTS, Moorman et al. (2016) consider context to also play a part in the strategy. Therefore the environment of a museum or art gallery can provide a contemplative and safe space to explore ideas, moving away from the hierarchical constraints of the classroom, lecture theatre or clinical area. This can free ideas and expressions, sometimes allowing discussion of complex and challenging topics such as ethical issues and diversity (see also

Moorman 2015, Moorman & Hensel 2016). The following excerpt from Moorman (2017, p. 169) describes how the questioning facilitator can move the active learning sessions along:

For example, when asked, "What is going on in this painting?" a student may reply, "I think that is a bird." The facilitator then asks, "What are you seeing that makes you think that is a bird?" The student may reply that the object has feathers, a beak, and wings, providing visual evidence to support his claim. The facilitator then paraphrases back, "So, based on the feathered structures at the object's side, and the attributes you described, you see this figure as a bird ... did I understand you correctly?" This allows the facilitator to demonstrate active learning and paraphrasing. Each time a student responds, the facilitator paraphrases back what he or she understood the student to say. Each time, the student has the opportunity to agree or to clarify.

This method could also be applied to your personal learning approach and, as with Action Learning, can be a useful method to apply when developing others or developing your own facilitation skills. As with Action Learning, the role of the facilitator is important – steering but not contributing to the ideas, emphasising and reiterating what the individual says, which is a powerful reinforcement of their ideas and prompts them to stop and think about what they have conveyed, to justify and clarify, and to think further about the image on a deeper level.

Try Reflective Activity 10.3 to practise this method. Having a trusted colleague or friend to apply this to will allow you to consider your ideas and form connections. Ideally a facilitator is needed; however you can begin to explore the effectiveness of this approach without one. You may want to explore your individual leadership, your team or your organisation, or skills that are associated with leadership, such as communication, creating a vision, emotional intelligence, compassion and values.

Reflective Activity: 10.3

Using this on a personal level, focusing on leadership and using the question prompts above, look at a painting of an artist you like. Alternatively, go to a museum or gallery and find an artwork you would like to explore. If you don't have access to this kind of venue, look for an artwork online or in a book. You could use a well-known image such as a work by Monet, Van Gogh or Hockney. Thinking in terms of leadership, consider the following:

- What is going on in this painting? Write this down if you are doing this individually and read it back.
- What are you seeing that makes you say that? Look at the image again and describe what has made you think about it as a representation of leadership.
- What more can you find? Try to think on a deeper level; think of experiences that may have motivated you, or maybe a critical event (as discussed in Chapter 4).

Identify two ideas or connections you would like to explore on a deeper level. What is the evidence around them, and are you able to explore them on a deeper reflexive level to take your development further?

10.5   STORYTELLING

Storytelling has been around as long as humans, conveying traditions, communicating and documenting events, exploring imagination and vision. In healthcare, storytelling has had a recent boost in significance through the use of patient stories, films and documentaries about the healthcare system, and as documentary evidence in significant events such as the COVID-19 pandemic. Sometimes it is hugely powerful and provides impetus for change (Wilson 2022). More widely, storytelling has always had emotional impact, providing meaning to experiences; and this emotional element makes a story powerful, creating meaning connection and knowledge (Egan & Judson 2015, Asma 2017).

Leaders who can craft their storytelling can engage their followers and audience, innovate and inspire, and convey their vision clearly (Judson 2023). As Conrad states (2016, p. 44), "Good leaders know stories can capture imaginations, illustrate ideas, arouse passions, and inspire creativity in ways that go far beyond the presentation of facts and data." Wenger (1999) links imagination to belonging; and, through storytelling, you can create shared meanings and encourage collaborative progress. You may read in the leadership literature, or hear when leaders talk about the need for change, the term 'changing the narrative'. When cultural change is required, and this can be applied to positive and negative circumstances, changing the story or changing the words used can be a powerful way to inspire change both for individuals and for organisations.

Personal leadership stories

There are many ways to use storytelling in leadership. For your own leadership development you might want to consider your personal story, divide it into chapters and plan out what

---

Reflective Activity: 10.4

Create your leadership story by thinking about and writing down responses to the following prompts:

- What is Chapter 1 in your leadership story? What was the significant event, who was involved in your story, what were your priorities and values, what motivated you?
- What came next? Using the preceding aspects, divide these significant areas into chapters. You can write as many as you want.
- When you reach the present time, think about the key learning from these chapters. What would you consider doing differently, what important insights have you gained?
- In terms of aspects of leadership, what were your strengths – when you communicated well, when you influenced, when you made decisive decisions, when you created impetus or effectively managed a team or a change? Write these into your story as reflections.
- Now think about where you are now in your leadership. How confident are you in your leadership? What do you need to drive your leadership forward? How can you get there? Begin to write the next chapter with these questions in mind; plot out your future leadership plan.
- In time you can revisit your story and planning chapter to see whether it needs rewriting and plan the next chapter in advance.

will come next. We very rarely reflect on our own lives in depth, and it can help to think about aspects of your leadership in terms of your story. By setting it out in this way, you can begin to gain insight into aspects that might influence where you are in your career and in your leadership. Examples could include how your priorities, values and motivations have an impact and how they change over time; and how they influenced your choices in life and in your career.

Storytelling as a leader

There are many ways in which storytelling can be used to inspire others and, as a leader, you can consider how this can have an impact on those you are leading. You could compile a collection of stories for different requirements, tailored to the motivating factors needed or the intended message. You might also want to tell your own leadership story to inspire.

Reflective Activity: 10.5

Poems and novels can also be powerful for inspiring others. You could relate or read a poem or story to begin a team meeting or training session. There are many poems and novels that tap into the emotions and can be inspiring. Consider the following passage from *The Celtic Twilight*, a series of stories by W.B.Yeats (2014 [1893]). What does it mean to you?

> The things a man has heard and seen are threads of life, and if he pull them carefully from the confused distaff of memory, any who will can weave them into whatever garments of belief please them best. … Hope and Memory have one daughter and her name is Art.

Historic tales of leadership can also be impactful, such as the story of Sir Ernest Shackleton, related in *Shackleton's Way: Leadership Lessons from the Great Antarctic Explorer* (Morrell & Capparell 2017). A tale of both success and failure, the narrative sets out the expedition of the *Endurance* in 1914–1916 and Shackleton's leadership approach in the face of adversity. A glimpse into his thirst for adventure is found in a letter to his wife on page 1: "I love the fight and when things [are] easy, I hate it."

The book tells of the lessons learnt and of Shackleton's influence; how he changed the way his men saw him and inspired them to keep going during the most hopeless of times, as evidenced by quotes from his crew on *Endurance* (Morrell & Capparell 2017, p. 13):

> I do not think there is any doubt that we all owe our lives to his leadership and his power of making a loyal and coherent party out of rather diverse elements. (Reginald W. James, physicist)

> No matter what turns up, he is always ready to alter his plans and make fresh ones, and in the meantime laughs, jokes and enjoys a joke with anyone, and in his way keeps everyone's spirits up. (Frank Worsley, Captain)

Think about an historical figure you admire, one who inspires you and demonstrates great leadership. You could choose someone from your profession, or a political figure or someone who had little recognition while alive but has since been champion of a cause. Read their story. Consider what their greatest strength was in leadership, and how you might use their story to inspire others.

Some organisations encourage staff to tell their own stories, record them and share them widely. In structuring stories there are some key tips to help create impact and make them memorable:

- Anecdotes and narratives that tell of successes and failures across careers can be impactful, with key learning points to highlight both.
- Stories that connect values to the profession or organisation using case studies and examples can reinforce aims and key messages.
- Stories that use examples of work culture can relate information and prompt others to think about the culture they work in.
- Narratives that inform and share knowledge can be effective ways of ensuring everyone is aware of particular topics.
- Stories of teams, both positive and negative, can inspire change or bring shared team goals together.

10.6 JOURNALING

Journaling is usually associated with a personal record of daily activities and thoughts. Leadership journaling is an extension and a more focused method, and can be effective for leadership development (Stanley 2022). This technique can encourage reflection and self-awareness. Taking time to write and reflect can help leaders move forward; so, rather than being introspective and stagnant in their leadership development, journaling can help leaders move things forward, explore new methods, opportunities and possibilities, and aid in critical thinking and problem solving. Taking time at the end of the day to reflect and write can also:

- Calm and solidify your thoughts, enable you to work through any issues or enable to you to confirm a successful day.
- Enable you to think about choices and decisions made and consider their impact.
- Build your story (add to your story as above).
- Improve your communication skills.
- Encourage critical thinking.
- Build self-confidence.
- Build emotional intelligence.

Where to start

Choose your format; you could buy a journal or decide to use an online format. It is important to choose something that doesn't feel like work or a work task; so, if your day involves using a computer all day, using a hardback notebook and a nice pen will feel less like work and more like a special form for reflection. Write down the following:

- Three or four things you feel you are good at as a leader.
- Three or four things you would like to improve as a leader.
- Three or four things you would like to try as a leader.

You can then reflect on these and begin to write down your thoughts and feelings. You could ask yourself a series of questions to start, such as: How would I describe my leadership approach? How do others see me as a leader? How do people respond to me as a leader?

Once you have written down your thoughts and feelings, consider what action you can take to progress in your leadership development. Write these down, along with any support or resources you might need to take such action. Then write down what you have learnt from the journal entry, including any realisations, such as achievements or areas for development, that have emerged from your reflection.

Journaling can also support coaching, and we considered coaching in Chapter 4 and how this can support your leadership development. Identifying goals, considering where you are in your leadership journey and identifying what you need to move forward can provide a self-coaching framework for your journaling. However it is important that your journaling does not become an opportunity for self-criticism; so, if you are thinking about things that have not gone well, ensure that you balance this with positives as there are always positives to be found. I have mentioned previously that it is often from mistakes and errors that we learn, so check in with your thoughts if you find you are being overly self-critical; remind yourself of the positive aspects of the day.

Try to form a journaling habit: set yourself ten minutes every day, whether before or after your workday, to write in your journal. Ask yourself the following:

- What am I curious about today, or what interested me about that event today?
- What do I want to learn more about today, or what did I learn about today?
- What surprised me?
- What does today mean for me as a leader?

With practice and some discipline you will find that journaling can organise your thoughts, calm your mind and help you set goals for your leadership path.

10.7   CONCLUSION

In this chapter I returned to reflection and presented some of the creative methods – such as journaling, visual thinking strategies and storytelling – that can support your leadership development over time. You may be drawn to more; however, I would encourage you to try at least one and see where it takes you.

REFERENCES

Asma, S. 2017. *The evolution of imagination*. Chicago: University of Chicago Press.

Collier, J., & Collier, M. 1986. *Visual anthropology*. Albuquerque: University of New Mexico Press.

Conrad, D. 2016. Inspire innovation by telling stories. *Journal of Leadership Studies*, 10, 44–45. https://doi.org/10.1002/jls.21440.

Cranston, J., & Kusanovich, K. 2014. How shall I act? Nurturing the dramatic and ethical imagination of educational leaders. *International Studies in Educational Administration*, 42(2), 45–62.

Dewey, J. 1980. *Art as experience*. New York: Perigee.

Egan, K., & Judson, G. 2015. *Imagination and the engaged learner: Cognitive tools for the classroom*. New York: Teachers College.

Ford, J., Harding, N., & Learmonth, M. 2008. *Leadership as identity: Constructions and deconstructions*. New York: Palgrave Macmillan.

Housen, A. 2002. Æsthetic thought, critical thinking and transfer. *Arts and Learning Research Journal*, 18(1), 99–131. https://vtshome.org/wp-content/uploads/2016/08/5%C3%86sthetic-Thought-Critical-Thinking-and-Transfer.pdf.

James, A.H. 2020. *Perceptions and experiences of leadership: A narrative inquiry of leadership in undergraduate nurse education*. Doctoral thesis, Cardiff University. http://orca.cardiff.ac.uk/id/eprint/140444.

James, A.H., Watkins, D., & Carrier, J. 2022. Perceptions and experiences of leadership in undergraduate nurse education: A narrative inquiry. *Nurse Education Today*, 111, 105313. https://doi.org/10.1016/j.nedt.2022.105313.

Judson, 2023. Cultivating leadership imagination with cognitive tools: An imagination focused approach to leadership education. *Journal of Research on Leadership Education*, 18(1), 40–62.

Klein, G. 1998. *Sources of power: How people make decisions*. Cambridge, MA: MIT Press.

Klenke, K. 2016. *Qualitative research in the study of leadership*. 2nd edn. Bingley: Emerald.

Moorman, M. 2015. The meaning of visual thinking strategies for nursing students. *Humanities*, 4(4), 748–759. https://doi.org/10.3390/h4040748.

Moorman, M. 2017. The use of visual thinking strategies and art to help nurses find their voices. *Creative Nursing*, 23(3), 167–171.

Moorman, M., & Hensel, D. 2016. Using visual thinking strategies in nursing education. *Nurse Educator*, 41(1), 5–6. http://dx.doi.org/10.1097/NNE.0000000000000185.

Moorman, M., Hensel, D., Decker, K., & Busby, K. 2016. Learning outcomes with visual thinking strategies in nursing education. *Nurse Education Today*, 51, 127–129. http://dx.doi.org/10.1016/j.nedt.2016.08.020.

Morrell, M., & Capparell, S. 2017. *Shackleton's way: Leadership lessons from the great Antarctic explorer*. London: Nicholas Brealey.

Stacey, R.D. 2010. *Complexity and organizational reality*. 2nd edn. London: Routledge.

Stanley, D. 2022. Creativity. In Stanley, D., Bennett, C.L., & James, A. (eds), *Clinical leadership in nursing and healthcare*. Hoboken, NJ: Wiley, pp. 205–226.

Vygotsky, L.S. 1993 [1978]. *The collected works of L.S. Vygotsky*. Vol. 2. New York: Plenum.

Wenger, E. 1999. *Communities of practice: Learning, meaning, and identity*. Cambridge: Cambridge University Press.

Wilson, M. 2022. *Arts for health: Storytelling*. Bingley: Emerald.

Yeats, W.B. 2014 [1893]. *Celtic twilight*. London: SMK Books.

CHAPTER 11

ACTION LEARNING FOR LEADERSHIP AND PROBLEM SOLVING

Alison H. James

11.1   WHAT IS ACTION LEARNING?

Here we will explore what Action Learning (AL) is and how it can support your leadership skills through the development of facilitation and problem solving techniques. I would define AL as an approach to learning and development based on reflection and experiential learning, drawing on experience, sharing knowledge and setting goals for action to problem solve and develop. Action Learning can aid the development of psychological support, emotional intelligence, team working and empowerment through an inclusive approach to problem-solving issues in the work environment. Leaders can demonstrate an inclusive, collective, compassionate leadership style through AL by inviting contributions, active listening, appreciating thoughts and agreeing actions, which allows for appreciation and ownership of achievements. This developmental approach to leadership has been shown to increase job satisfaction in the workplace, encourage innovation and creativity, and reduce psychological distress (Ahmed et al. 2021, James & Arnold 2022).

The concept of AL originates with Reg Revans (1980), a fascinating man with a strong value base. In his writing he often refers to ethical values and principles, respect for others and social responsibility, and his work on AL promoted inclusivity (Abbott & Taylor 2013). With a background in science research and then the coal industry, Revans became interested in education and development and creative solutions to problems in organisations. Acknowledging rapid change within organisations, he believed that people and organisations can thrive through maintaining the rate of *Learning* with the rate of *Change*. He therefore developed a formula that acknowledged two aspects of learning (L) – instructed learning programmed knowledge (P) and critical insight or reflection (Q). Using the formula L=P+Q, Revans explains that: "P is the concern of the traditional academy; Q is the field of action learning" (1980, p. 16).

This is similar to what we have discussed previously as critical thinking, reflection and reflexivity, recognising that, while knowledge can come from sources of theory and evidence, experience is also a key part of that knowledge building and critical thinking towards deeper learning. The principles of AL require identifying a *problem* rather than a *puzzle*. A 'puzzle' is easily solvable with the right resources, and does not require deeper thinking and learning. A 'problem' is more complex, and requires critical thinking and drawing on experience and resources, which may include evidence or theory.

While AL involves a group context and is a problem-solving method to encourage deep learning (Marquardt & Banks 2010), it has been used increasingly within healthcare, clinical practice and nursing and social care education to good effect (James & Stacey-Emile 2019). Using a questioning formula, AL can motivate and encourage sharing of problems, knowledge and ideas in a safe environment. The accepted ground rules of Action Learning Sets (ALS) establish trust and confidentiality within groups, which in turn can encourage openness and honesty, preparing the ground for moving forward and setting realistic goals (James & Stacey-Emile 2019).

An Action Learning Set consists of a group of people, usually a maximum of eight, who meet on a regular basis to introduce a problem or issue they wish to work through. The group can consist of different professions and positions. Members share ideas and develop individual goals through problem solving and action; individuals share their issue or what they wish to

DOI: 10.4324/9781003433354-13

achieve; and, with periods of reflection and thinking, members of the group will offer ideas and suggestions, sharing experience and knowledge and providing incremental steps forward for the individual to set actions and goals. It is an effective method for leaders to introduce into practice areas effectively for small groups, with the aid of a facilitator (Pedler & Abbott 2013, Christiansen et al. 2014).

The relationships formed within the process of an ALS can encourage collective growth and sharing of knowledge and experience, seeking problem solving, cooperative development of goals and acceptance of 'self' as leader (Rosser et al. 2017). During each ALS, previous goals are revisited and progress is reported; or, if further issues or problems have prohibited this, these can be addressed. It is very much an approach to problem solving over time, not based on impulse or urgency but allowing the process and individuals involved to set their pace and by taking action to ensure the change is embedded. I like to think of it as a Van Gogh approach (1882): "For the great doesn't happen through impulse alone and is a succession of little things that are brought together."

One advantage of AL is that, while it was originally developed as a face-to-face process, it is also effective when individuals are remote and can only meet via an online forum for example. During the COVID-19 pandemic, AL in healthcare was used to address complex issues and drive change (Papanagnou et al. 2022, James & Arnold 2022). As a timed and facilitated process, this also means its focused approach is well suited to the busy and time-starved health and care workforce. A sample framework for the ALS process is shown in Figure 11.1.

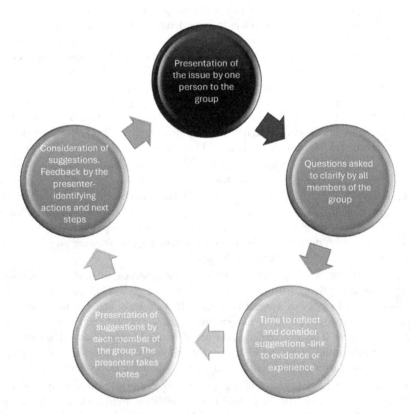

Figure 11.1 The Action Learning Set (ALS) process
Adapted from James and Stacey-Emile (2019).

11.2   CRITICAL ACTION LEARNING

Critical Action Learning (CAL) can be an effective process to help leaders focus their teams on prioritised goals. CAL involves collaboration and critical thinking; however it further explores relationship dynamics that may influence organisational culture and power structures. These can hinder teams from functioning effectively and positively, so CAL can support a more innovative and creative approach to working together (Pedler & Abbott 2013). Participants are required to agree to mutual respect, and must share core values for CAL to be effective, taking responsibility for action on agreed goals.

11.3   PERSONAL SKILLS FOR ALS

Whether you are participating in ALS or facilitating an ALS, there is a need for various skills associated with leadership. These include:

- Communication – being able to express ideas clearly and communicate effectively with others
- Active listening – listening with intent
- Problem solving – have a can-do attitude
- Critical thinking – the ability to question and be inquisitive
- Clarity of thought and focus – remaining focused on others' issues as well as your own
- Being non-judgemental
- Being observant – noticing group dynamics and stepping in if needed
- Inclusivity
- Emotional and social intelligence
- Trust and confidentiality – setting and keeping to the ground rules
- Being supportive and challenging
- Paraphrasing the message
- Valuing others' contributions
- Working with silence – pause for thought and reflection are needed.

Reflective Activity: 11.1

Visit the link below to Gwella, the leadership portal run by Health Education and Improvement Wales (HEIW), and listen to the talk on 'conscious listening'.

Consider why listening is important within Action Learning.

What are the challenges to 'conscious listening'?

https://nhswalesleadershipportal.heiw.wales/about-gwella.

Pedler and Abbott (2013) further consider the particular leadership skills AL can be helpful in supporting, including: collaboration; the ability to step back and see things in a new light based on other experiences; and the power to bring people together around a common cause. This points to working interprofessionally, and ALS is a good tool to break down professional tension and bring teams together. There is no space for hierarchy within AL. Indeed, it is important when creating an ALS that power and hierarchical positions do not influence the group dynamic, and the facilitator's role will include identifying any power plays within the group. The facilitator's main roles are to:

- **Be attentive** – invest in the process
- **Listen** – to help clarify
- **Empathise** – understand the challenges
- **Reflect** – to plan ahead and drive the learning
- **Question** – to help members find solutions
- **Respond** – have a range of options if the group is 'stuck'
- **Intervene** – if needed and if 'sabotaging' occurs
- **Feedback** – help learning and place value on contributions
- **Summarise** – recap, focus and ensure understanding and action

Asking questions to gain deeper insight might also be required to prompt the ALS members further, encourage the exchange of ideas, make the learning explicit and encourage risk in goal setting and action. These can be as simple as:

- What are you trying to do?
- What are the barriers?
- Who or what can help?

Values-based leadership styles, such as compassionate leadership (West 2021), sit well with the ethos of Action Learning by: encouraging self-awareness, emotional and social intelligence; supporting individuals to perform at their best and feel safe in their work environment; valuing individual strengths and contributions; promoting individual and team potential; and allowing each member to be heard and have a shared purpose to drive for effective and safe patient care. Box 11.1 presents a sample template in preparation for use with groups for ALS.

11.4 CONCLUSION

Action Learning is a process that addresses problems and issues, and here we have introduced the concept and discussed how it can support leadership development and be effective for leaders to use. As a process, its benefits include encouraging interdisciplinary working, collective learning and sharing, and using experience and critical thinking to set goals and take action.

Box 11.1   Action Learning template for ALS participants

Preparation: Please complete this in advance and bring it to the Action Learning Set (ALS).
You can use this to make notes for suggestions you find helpful and to set your actions for
the next ALS. Keep this for your own reflective log and evidence of learning.

1. Briefly describe the issue/problem you would like support with.

2. Why is it important for your project?

3. What issues would you like to address first?

4. What suggestions have been most helpful?

After the ALS session, write down up to **three** next action steps you will now take to
move the project forward. What are my next steps?

Reflective Activity: 11.2

Consider the challenges of facilitating an Action Learning Set.

What leadership skills might you need to overcome these challenges?

How might you approach a situation where one person is dominating the conversation?

How can you ensure that every person is heard and contributes to the group?

How will you know if all members of the group are actively engaging in the ALS
process?

What would you do to encourage engagement?

REFERENCES

Abbott, C., & Taylor, P. 2013. *Action learning in social work*. London: Sage.

Ahmed, F., Zhao, F., Faraz, N.A., & Qin, Y.J. 2021. How inclusive leadership paves way for psychological well-being of employees during trauma and crisis: A three-wave longitudinal mediation study. *Journal of Advanced Nursing*, 77(2), 819–831. doi:10.1111/jan.14637.

Christiansen, A., Prescott, T., & Ball, J. 2014. Learning in action: Developing safety improvement capabilities through action learning. *Nurse Education Today*, 34(2), 243–247.

James, A.H., & Arnold, H. 2022. Using coaching and action learning to support staff leadership development. *Nursing Management*, 29(3), 32–40. https://doi.org/10.7748/nm.2022.e2040.

James, A.H., & Stacey-Emile, G. 2019. Action Learning: Staff development, implementing change, interdisciplinary working, and leadership. *Nursing Management*, 26(3), 36–41. doi:10.7748/nm. 2019.e1841.

Marquardt, M., & Banks, S. 2010. Theory to practice: Action learning. *Advances in Developing Human Resources*, 12(2), 159–162.

Papanagnou, D., Watkins, K., Lundgren, H., Alcid, G.A., Ziring, D., & Marsick, V.J. 2022. Informal and incidental learning in the clinical learning environment: Learning through complexity and uncertainty during Covid-19. *Academic Medicine*, 97(8), 1137–1143. https://doi.org/10.1097/ACM.0000000000004717.

Pedler, M., & Abbott, C. 2013. *Facilitating action learning: A practitioner's guide*. Maidenhead: Open University Press.

Revans, R. 1980. *Action learning: New techniques for management*. London: Blond & Briggs.

Rosser, E., Grey, R., Neal, D., Reeve, J., Smith, C., & Valentine, J. 2017. Supporting clinical leadership through action: The nurse consultant role. *Journal of Clinical Nursing*, 26(23–24), 4768–4776.

Van Gogh, V. 1882. Letter number: 274. From Vincent van Gogh to Theo van Gogh. The Hague, Sunday, 22 October 1882. Van Gogh Museum of Amsterdam. Van Gogh Letters Project database. https://vangoghletters.org/vg/letters/let274/letter.html (Accessed: 16 August 2024).

West, M.A. 2021. *Compassionate leadership: Sustaining wisdom, humanity and presence in health and social care*. London: Swirling Leaf Press.

INDEX

Note: **Bold** page numbers refer to tables; *italic* page numbers refer to figures.

Printed in the United States
by Baker & Taylor Publisher Services